The Primary FRCA Structured Oral Examination Study Guide 2

KATE McCOMBE MBBS MRCP FRCA
Specialist Registrar Anaesthetics
Poole Hospital, Dorset

LARA WIJAYASIRI MBBS BSC FRCA
Specialist Registrar Anaesthetics
St George's Hospital, London

and

AMISH PATEL MBBS FRCA
Consultant, Intensive Care Medicine & Anaesthetics
The Royal Surrey County Hospital, Guildford

Foreword by

DAVID BOGOD
Consultant Anaesthetist
Editor-in-Chief, Anaesthesia

Radcliffe Publishing
Oxford • New York

Radcliffe Publishing Ltd
St Marks House
Shepherdess Walk
London
N1 7BQ

www.radcliffe-oxford.com

Electronic catalogue and worldwide online ordering facility.

British Library Cataloguing in Publication Data

A catalogue record for this book is available from the British Library.

ISBN–13: 978 184619 434 4

The paper used for the text pages of this book is FSC certified. FSC (The Forest Stewardship Council) is an international network to promote responsible management of the world's forests.

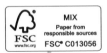

Typeset by Pindar NZ, Auckland, New Zealand
Printed and bound by TJI Digital, Padstow, Cornwall, UK

Contents

Foreword

Whatever happened to the Senior Registrar? When I was a first-year trainee, we knew where to go for help, whether with a difficult case, an obstreperous colleague or an upcoming exam. The consultants were too remote and, more importantly, not always in possession of the latest facts. The SR, omnipresent and omnipotent, was a god-like creature; men wanted to be like them, women wanted to bear their children. A study published when I was in my second year of training showed that anaesthetic SRs had the lowest rate of critical incidents of any grade of anaesthetists, despite looking after the sickest patients; none of my SHO colleagues was in the least bit surprised.

While the title may have passed into history, the spirit of the Senior Registrar is alive and kicking in the forms of Drs McCombe, Wijayasiri and Patel (although Dr Patel has now made it to the top). They all passed their FRCA Primary first time and then – having ticked off the rest of the exam in a similarly airy fashion – immediately settled down to help others do the same. This book is the result.

What sets this book apart from others purporting to smooth your passage through the Primary? The authors have paid scrupulous attention to the Royal College's guide to the exam, covering not only the topics listed in the current edition, but also those in the previous edition, many of which still come up in the Structured Oral Examination (SOE). Rather than cherry-picking a number of topics from the long College syllabus, they have dealt with each and every one of them, from as many different angles as they could imagine the examiners finding.

As well as using this scrupulously comprehensive approach, the authors have included vignettes on those critical incidents such as blood transfusion error and local anaesthetic toxicity (*Study Guide 2*) which are likely to form part of the clinical SOE. A section on 'special patient groups' (*Study Guide 2*) covers topics such as diabetes, neonates, Jehovah's Witnesses and obese patients, in a format which allows the candidate to easily incorporate the information into problems posed during the SOE. The pharmacology section (*Study Guide 1*) includes 'spider diagrams' for all commonly used drugs in anaesthesia; the consistency of this unique format makes it easier to find and absorb information quickly in those angina-inducing hours before the MCQ or SOE. The 'physics' section (*Study Guide 2*) covers all those topics which the consultants have either long-forgotten or – perhaps even worse – have made their pet interest upon which they can expound throughout a long plastics list. Here, everything is handled in a page or two of short notes; information-rich and waffle-poor, these short vignettes are just what are needed as the exam date looms nearer.

In short, if you are not lucky enough to be working in the same hospital as the authors, and can't approach them for exam practice (or even if you can), then this book is an essential companion and a true *vade mecum*. Look it up – a bit of Latin can still impress the examiners!

David Bogod
Consultant Anaesthetist, Nottingham
Editor-in-Chief, *Anaesthesia*
January 2010

Preface

During our revision for the primary exam we were advised that the best way to ensure success in the structured oral examination (SOE) was to prepare answers to all of the questions in the back of *The Royal College of Anaesthetists Guide to the FRCA Examination, The Primary*. Undoubtedly, this was excellent advice but it proved an enormous task and one we simply did not have time to complete before our own exams. However, once they were over, we began to answer all those questions in the hope that this might help others to prepare for the Primary, or for the basic science component of the Final FRCA. Finally then, here is the result: the book we wish we'd had.

The Primary FRCA Structured Oral Examination Study Guide provides answers to the questions regularly posed by the examiners. We have not attempted to write the next great anaesthetic textbook, but rather to collate information and deliver it in a relevant and user-friendly layout to make your exam preparation a little easier.

In the SOE itself, each topic will be examined for approximately five minutes. Many of these answers contain much more information than could reasonably be expected of you in that time; however, we have tried to cover several angles of questioning.

We have included the usual chapters on physiology, pharmacology (*Study Guide 1*) and physics (*Study Guide 2*) and, in addition, have written a section on patients who present the anaesthetist with unique problems, 'special patient groups' (*Study Guide 2*). These patients tend to appear in the clinical SOE before some terrible 'critical incident' befalls them. Again, we have included a section addressing the 'critical incidents' beloved of the examiner, with advice as to how to approach them in the SOE (*Study Guide 2*).

There is a unique pharmacology section including information on drugs commonly examined presented in a spider diagram layout. These extremely visual learning aids allowed us to revise the drugs in the necessary detail, and helped us to recall the information even under the acute stress of the exam. We hope you find them just as useful.

We wish you every success in what is undoubtedly a rigorous exam. We believe the key to this success is to practise presenting the knowledge that you already have, logically and concisely. The only way to do this is to practise speaking, even though the possibility of exposing any ignorance is daunting. The more you talk, the more you will cover, and every question is so much easier to answer in the exam if you have already had a dress rehearsal. We hope this book will help you in your preparations.

Good luck!

Lara Wijayasiri
Kate McCombe
Amish Patel
January 2010

'Examinations are formidable even to the best prepared,
for the greatest fool may ask more than the wisest man can answer.'

CC Colton

To Andrew, who makes me believe anything is possible.
Kate McCombe

To Amish, my husband and best friend, thank you
for helping me achieve this.
Lara Wijayasiri

To Lara, my wife and soulmate.
Amish Patel

Contributors

Dr Barbara Lattuca MBBCh MRCP FRCA
Specialist Registrar Anaesthetics
St George's Hospital, London

Pharmacology
➤ Drugs and the kidney
➤ Inhalational anaesthetic agents (volatile agents)

Dr Mark Wyldbore MBBS BSc(Hons) RAMC
ST4 Anaesthetics
St George's Hospital, London

Pharmacology
➤ Drugs and the liver
➤ Total intravenous anaesthesia
➤ Anticoagulants

The Primary FRCA Examination

The Primary FRCA is divided into two parts: a Multiple Choice Question (MCQ) paper followed by an Objective Structured Clinical Exam (OSCE) and a Structured Oral Examination (SOE). The MCQ paper takes place on one day (at various locations throughout the UK) and some weeks later the OSCE and SOE take place together at the Royal College of Anaesthetists in London. There are three exam sittings per year.

GENERAL GUIDELINES

MCQ

➤ You are allowed a maximum of five attempts at the MCQ examination (this also applies to those candidates who have failed the examination under previous eligibility criteria).
➤ The MCQ paper must be passed in order to progress to the OSCE and SOE.

OSCE and SOE

➤ The OSCE and SOE are now marked as stand-alone examinations.
➤ At the first attempt, the OSCE and SOE must be taken at the same sitting. If you pass one component but fail the other, you have only to re-take the failed component. However, if you fail both components, you must continue taking them together until you have passed either one or both. You may attempt each part of the examination no more than four times.

EXAMINATION AND MARKING STRUCTURE

MCQ (3 hours)

➤ The paper consists of 90 questions covering three subsections: approximately 30 questions on pharmacology, 30 on physiology and 30 questions on physics and clinical measurement (including statistics and data interpretation).
➤ One mark is allocated for each correct answer.
➤ The paper is positively marked.
➤ The pass mark is expected to be approximately 80%.
➤ Your performance in each of the three subsections is taken into consideration; those who perform very poorly in one or more subsections will fail the MCQ regardless of a cumulative mark higher than the pass mark.
➤ The single best answer (SBA) format for some questions will be introduced from 2011.

OSCE (1 hour 50 minutes)

➤ The OSCE consists of 18 stations, of which only 16 are counted towards your examination score.
➤ Two 'trial stations' are included in the 18 in order to test new questions, but neither

the examiners nor the candidates will know which stations these are. The results of these two will not contribute towards your final mark.

➤ The stations comprise resuscitation, technical skills, anatomy (which may include a general procedure), history taking, physical examination, communication skills, X-ray interpretation, anaesthetic equipment, monitoring equipment, measuring equipment and anaesthetic hazards.

➤ Some stations may involve the use of a simulator.

➤ Each station is marked out of 20, with the pass mark for each station being predetermined by the examiners by modified Angoff referencing.

➤ Your aggregate score (the sum of the marks obtained at each station) will be calculated and either a 'pass' or 'fail' awarded depending on your overall performance.

SOE 1 (30 minutes)

➤ Two examiners conduct each SOE. You will be questioned by the first examiner on one subject for 15 minutes, while the other observes and marks your performance. The examiners then trade places and the previously silent one examines the second subject, while his partner observes.

➤ In each 15 minutes, you will be asked questions on three different topics, relating to the subject being examined. In SOE 1, these subjects are pharmacology and physiology and biochemistry.

➤ A score of 0, 1 or 2 (fail, borderline or pass) will be allocated per question by each examiner. This means that the maximum total score for SOE 1 is 24 (there are two examiners, each marking a total of six questions, each of which can achieve a maximum mark of two).

SOE 2 (30 minutes)

➤ The format of SOE 2 is as described above.

➤ 15 minutes will be spent asking three questions on physics, clinical measurement, equipment and safety and the other 15 asking three questions on clinical topics, including a problem-based scenario (critical incident).

➤ The marking of SOE 2 is identical to that of SOE 1.

➤ The marks achieved for both SOE 1 and SOE 2 are combined together to give an aggregate score. The maximum total score achievable is 48. The candidate will need a score of 37 or more in order to pass.

For up-to-date information on the examination format and syllabus, visit the Royal College website: www.rcoa.ac.uk.

1

Pharmacology

GENERIC DRUG DIAGRAM

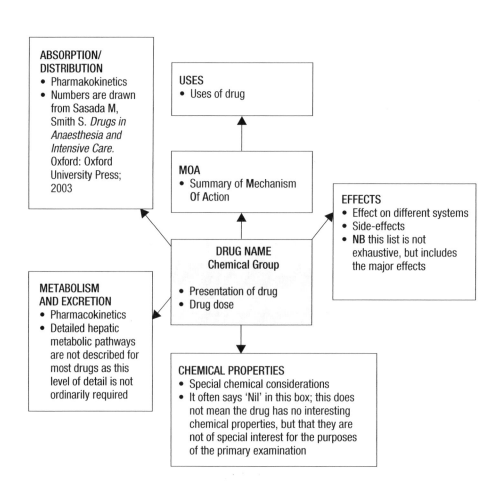

**ABSORPTION/
DISTRIBUTION**
- Pharmakokinetics
- Numbers are drawn from Sasada M, Smith S. *Drugs in Anaesthesia and Intensive Care.* Oxford: Oxford University Press; 2003

USES
- Uses of drug

MOA
- Summary of Mechanism Of Action

EFFECTS
- Effect on different systems
- Side-effects
- NB this list is not exhaustive, but includes the major effects

**DRUG NAME
Chemical Group**

- Presentation of drug
- Drug dose

**METABOLISM
AND EXCRETION**
- Pharmacokinetics
- Detailed hepatic metabolic pathways are not described for most drugs as this level of detail is not ordinarily required

CHEMICAL PROPERTIES
- Special chemical considerations
- It often says 'Nil' in this box; this does not mean the drug has no interesting chemical properties, but that they are not of special interest for the purposes of the primary examination

CHAPTER 1

Receptors

Define 'receptor' and 'ligand'

Receptors are proteins, usually integral to the cell membrane, with selective ligand-binding sites.

A **ligand** is any substance able to bind to a receptor and bring about biological change within the cell. A ligand may be capable of binding to more than one receptor and exerting different effects at each one.

What governs drug-receptor interactions?

The **law of mass action** governs drug-receptor interactions and so the rate of interaction is proportional to the concentration of drug and receptor. It is a specific, dose-dependent and saturatable interaction.

What are the different classes of receptors?

TABLE 1.1 Receptor classes

Receptor	Ligand-gated ion channel receptor	G-protein coupled receptor	Tyrosine kinase linked receptor	Intracellular nuclear receptors
Location	Membrane	Membrane	Membrane	Cytosol
Effector	Channel	Enzyme/Channel	Tyrosine kinase	Gene transcription
Coupling	Direct	G-protein	Direct	via DNA
Speed	Milliseconds	Seconds	Minutes	Hours
Examples	nAChR GABA$_A$	mAChR Adrenoceptors	Insulin receptor	Thyroxine receptor Steroid receptor

What are the main mechanisms of receptor action?

➤ **Altered ion permeability:**
  - Acetylcholine (ACh) binds to the 2 α subunits of the pentameric nicotinic acetylcholine receptor (nAChR), causing a conformational change, which opens a central pore allowing an influx of Na$^+$ ions, which leads to cell depolarisation.
  - Benzodiazepines bind to a specific site on the GABA$_A$ receptor (nAChR), causing a conformational change, which opens a central pore allowing an influx of Cl$^-$ ions which leads to cell hyperpolarisation.

➤ **Intermediate (secondary) messengers:**
  - There are several types of secondary messengers including cyclic adenosine monophosphate (cAMP), cyclic guanosine monophosphate (cGMP), inositol triphosphate (IP$_3$), diacylglycerol (DAG) and calcium ions (Ca^{2+}).
  - These are involved in signal transduction and signal amplification and the rate of production of these second messengers is altered by a ligand binding to a G-protein coupled receptor (GPCR).

- They have a diverse effect on the cell by activation of protein kinases and modulation of calcium channels.
- cAMP is activated by Gs proteins (e.g. via stimulation of β adrenoceptors and glucagon receptors).
- cAMP is inhibited by Gi proteins (e.g. via stimulation of α_2 adrenoceptors and opioid receptors).
- IP_3 and DAG are activated by Gq proteins (e.g. via stimulation of α_1 adrenoceptors and muscarinic acetylcholine receptors).
- cGMP is activated by nitric oxide.
➤ **Regulation of gene transcription:**
- These receptors are located intracellularly and are targeted by lipid-soluble ligands, typically hormones (e.g. thyroxine and steroids) which can easily diffuse into the cell.
- Once in the cytosol, the ligands bind with receptors and then the ligand-receptor complex enters the nucleus, alters DNA transcription and therefore protein synthesis.
- This system operates over a matter of hours, which explains why it takes 6 to 8 hours to achieve a clinical response following hydrocortisone administration in acute asthma.

What is the structure of the G-protein coupled receptor (GPCR)?
➤ GPCR consist of seven α helices, which span the cell membrane forming an extracellular site (where the ligand binds) and an intracellular site (where the G-protein attaches).
➤ Each GPCR can be associated with up to a hundred G-proteins, which promotes signal amplification.

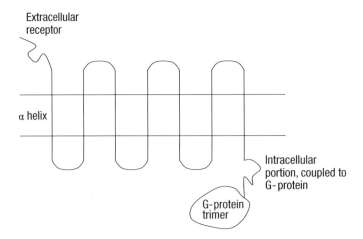

FIGURE 1.2 Schematic representation of a G-protein coupled receptor

What are G-proteins?
➤ G-proteins (or GTP-binding proteins) are regulatory proteins, which couple the activation of a surface receptor to the activation of an intracellular enzyme (e.g. adenylate cyclase) so that a secondary messenger can be produced (e.g. cAMP), allowing signal transduction and amplification to occur.

➤ They are heterotrimeric proteins (i.e. they consist of α, β and γ subunits which join together to form a trimer).

Which different types of G-proteins are there?
➤ The main types of G-proteins are the 'stimulatory' (i.e. Gs and Gq) and the 'inhibitory' (i.e. Gi) proteins.
➤ Gs proteins stimulate adenylate cyclase, causing a rise in cAMP (e.g. β adrenoceptors and glucagon receptor).
➤ Gq proteins stimulate phospholipase C, causing a rise in IP_3 and DAG (e.g. α_1 adrenoceptor and mAChR).
➤ Gi proteins inhibit adenylate cyclase, causing a fall in cAMP (e.g. α_2 adrenoceptors and opioid receptors).

What happens when a GPCR is activated?
➤ When a ligand binds to the extracellular site of a GPCR, it causes a GTP molecule to bind to the intracellular α subunit of the G-protein trimer.
➤ This causes a conformational change within the trimer resulting in its separation from the receptor and dissociation into a βγ and an α-GTP complex.
➤ The α-GTP complex then goes on to activate (or inhibit) the various enzymes systems (e.g. adenylate cyclase, guanylate cyclase and phospholipase C) resulting in the production of the secondary messengers.
➤ The α subunit has intrinsic GTPase activity and so it converts the GTP into GDP.
➤ Once the α subunit is bound only to GDP, it rejoins the βγ units to return to its resting state. The reformed G-protein trimer reattaches to the intracellular portion of the receptor and the receptor system is ready to be stimulated once again.

CHAPTER 2

Mechanism of drug action

How do drugs work?

Drugs produce their effects by acting on numerous different systems within the body. Below is a list of the effecter sites at which drugs act, along with some clinical examples.

Receptors
- Ligand-gated ion channels
  - Suxamethonium is an agonist at nAChR while rocuronium is an antagonist.
  - Diazepam is an agonist at $GABA_A$ receptors while flumazenil is an antagonist.
- G-protein coupled receptors
  - Dobutamine is an agonist at β-adrenoceptors while atenolol is an antagonist.
  - Morphine is an agonist at opioid receptors while naloxone is an antagonist.
- Tyrosine kinase receptors
  - Insulin is an agonist at insulin receptors.
- Intracellular receptors
  - Hydrocortisone is an agonist at steroid receptors.

Ion channels
- Lignocaine blocks the fast Na^+ channels.
- Verapamil blocks L-type Ca^{2+} channels.

Enzymes
- Neostigmine inhibits acetylcholinesterase.
- Aspirin inhibits cyclo-oxygenase 1 and 2.

Hormones
- Carbimazole reduced thyroxine production.
- Metformin increases insulin production.

Neurotransmitters
- Ephedrine increases presynaptic noradrenaline release.
- Amitriptyline and cocaine reduce noradrenaline reuptake.

Transport systems
- Digoxin inhibits the cardiac Na^+/K^+ ATPase pump.
- Furosemide inhibits the $Na^+/K^+/2Cl^-$ ATPase pump in the loop of Henle.

Physicochemical
- Sugammadex chelates rocuronium.
- Antacids neutralise gastric acids.

CHAPTER 3

Drug interactions

What is a drug interaction?
- A drug interaction occurs when the action of one drug is altered by the concurrent or prior administration of another drug.
- It is estimated that one in six drug charts contain a significant drug interaction and this is becoming increasingly more important as many patients are on multiple drugs, some of which can interfere with anaesthetic agents.

How can drug interactions be classified?
- **Physicochemical** drug interactions occur due to the physical properties of the drugs themselves.
- **Pharmacokinetic** drug interactions occur when one drug alters the way in which the body handles another.
- **Pharmacodynamic** drug interactions occur when the action of one drug is altered by the administration of another.

Give examples of physicochemical drug interactions you may encounter
Some drug interactions are clinically useful:
- **Chelation**
  - Sugammadex and rocuronium.
- **Neutralisation**
  - Heparin and protamine.

Others occur inadvertently with undesirable effects:
- **Precipitation**
  - Thiopentone (weak acid) and suxamethonium (weak base).
- **Adsorption**
  - Halothane dissolving into rubber.

Give examples of pharmacokinetic drug interactions
These drug interactions can affect drug absorption, distribution, metabolism and excretion.
- Absorption
  - Adrenaline administered with local anaesthetics reduces absorption of the local anaesthetic by causing local vasoconstriction.
- Distribution
  - Aspirin (80% plasma protein bound) displaces warfarin (97% plasma protein bound) from plasma proteins, thereby increasing the unbound fraction of warfarin and increasing the risk of bleeding.
- Metabolism
  - Phenytoin, carbamazepine, rifampicin and barbiturates induce hepatic enzymes, which results in the accelerated breakdown of drugs metabolised by these enzymes.
  - Omeprazole and cimetidine inhibit hepatic enzymes, reducing the breakdown of drugs metabolised by these enzymes.

➤ Excretion
  ● Alkalinising the urine increases the renal excretion of salicylates.

Give examples of pharmacodynamic drug interactions

➤ **Summation** occurs when the action of two or more drugs is additive (i.e. 1+1=2):
  ● nitrous oxide and inhalational anaesthetic agents.
➤ **Synergism** occurs when the combined action of two or more drugs is greater than the sum of their individual effects (i.e. 1+1 > 2):
  ● propofol and remifentanil.
➤ **Potentiation** occurs when the action of one drug is increased by the administration of another drug:
  ● probenecid increases the action of penicillin by reducing its renal excretion.
➤ **Antagonism** occurs when the action of one drug is blocked or reversed by another drug (i.e. 1+1=0):
  ● morphine and naloxone.

CHAPTER 4

Drug absorption and bioavailability

What factors influence drug absorption?

Drug absorption describes the passage of a drug into the bloodstream from its route of administration. Factors influencing this are as follows:

➤ **Route of administration**
➤ **Particle size**
➤ **pKa and ionisation**
➤ **Lipid solubility:** The more lipid-soluble a drug, the more readily it can cross the phospholipid bilayer of cells, and the faster it is absorbed.
➤ **Concentration gradient:** The higher the concentration gradient between the lumen containing the 'drug load' and the cells into which it is diffusing, the faster it will be absorbed.
➤ **Other factors:** Bacterial overgrowth will reduce drug absorption and some drugs will be affected by intake of other substances, e.g. milk chelates tetracycline antibiotics and so decreases their availability for absorption.

How can manufacturers alter rate of drug absorption?

Most drugs are taken orally and pass from the mouth into the aqueous and acidic environment of the stomach. Here they may dissolve and cross into the cells lining the stomach. Dissolution and absorption can be altered by the manufacturers in several ways:

➤ **Particle size:** The larger the particle size (molecular weight) of the drug, the more slowly it will dissolve.
➤ **Compounds used:** Different compounds dissolve at different rates. Modified-release or slow-release drugs can improve the drug profile, minimising peaks and troughs in plasma concentration. Patient compliance improves with less frequent dosing.
➤ **Coating the tablet:** Enteric coating does not dissolve in acid conditions and therefore the drug will pass to the basic intestine before dissolving.

What are the available routes for drug administration?

➤ Transdermal
➤ Intra-nasal
➤ Sublingual
➤ Buccal
➤ Tracheal
➤ Intravenous (bioavailability is taken as 1.0 or 100%)
➤ Intramuscular
➤ Epidural
➤ Subarachnoid
➤ Rectal
➤ Vaginal

What is pKa and how does this influence drug absorption?
➤ The Ka is the dissociation constant and it describes how readily an acid in solution gives up its hydrogen ions to a base.
➤ It describes the ratio of the products of the reaction, to the concentration of the initial reactants.
➤ It is written:

$$Ka = \frac{[A^-][H^+]}{[HA]}$$

Where HA is the acid; A^- is its conjugate base (i.e. the product that is now able to accept protons) and H^+ its proton. The higher the value of Ka, the more readily the acid gives up its proton and dissociates.
➤ The pKa is the acid dissociation constant, and is defined as $-\log_{10}$ Ka.
➤ At pH < pKa, acidic drugs become less ionised:

$$HA \rightleftharpoons H^+ + A^-$$

Putting the acidic drug in a more acidic environment raises H^+ concentration and so drives the equation to the left.
➤ At pH < pKa, basic drugs become more ionised as they accept protons:

$$B + H^+ \rightleftharpoons BH^+$$

Putting a basic drug in an acidic environment drives the equation to the right as the base (B) 'accepts' the protons.
➤ Drugs cross membranes in the un-ionised state and so their pKa and the pH of the surrounding environment affect their rate of absorption. Hence, acidic drugs will be more readily absorbed in the highly acidic stomach, whereas basic drugs are better absorbed in the intestine where pH is higher.

What is the Henderson–Hasselbalch equation and how is it useful in predicting drug absorption?
➤ The Henderson–Hasselbalch equation describes the derivation of pH as a measure of acidity. pH is calculated using the pKa and the equation can be expressed in two ways:

$$pH = pKa + \log \frac{[\text{conjugate base}]}{[\text{acid}]}$$

$$pH = pKa + \log \frac{[A^-]}{[HA]}$$

Where pKa is $-\log (Ka)$.

➤ Using the non-specific acid–base reaction: $HA + H_2O \rightleftharpoons A^- + H_3O^+$
pKa can be substituted into the equation, to give the Henderson–Hasselbalch equation:

$$-\log (Ka) = -\log \frac{[H_3O^+][A^-]}{[HA]}$$

➤ This is used to calculate:
• pH of a solution
• pH at which an equation is in equilibrium (i.e. the pKa)
• proportions of ionised and un-ionised drug in a solution at a given pH.

Define bioavailability
➤ Bioavailability describes the fraction of the drug administered that reaches the bloodstream.
➤ If a drug is given intravenously it is introduced straight into the bloodstream and is said to have a bioavailability of 1 or 100%.
➤ For drugs given orally, the bioavailability is calculated by comparing the plasma concentration of the drug when administered orally to the plasma concentration when it is administered intravenously. This is achieved by comparing the area under the curve (AUC) of the two conditions:

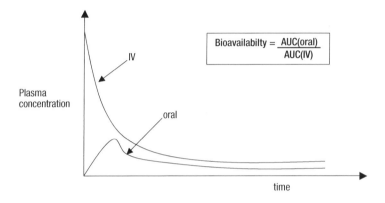

$$\text{Bioavailabilty} = \frac{\text{AUC(oral)}}{\text{AUC(IV)}}$$

GRAPH 1.3 Plasma concentrations of a drug administered intravenously and orally

What is first pass metabolism?
➤ This refers to the process by which drugs absorbed from the gastrointestinal tract enter the hepatic portal circulation and are carried to the liver. The liver then metabolises the drug such that only a fraction of the original dose is returned to the systemic circulation.
➤ Drugs that undergo extensive first pass metabolism have low oral bioavailability and it may be necessary to find an alternative route of administration which allows the drug to enter the systemic circulation directly.

Can you give examples of drugs which undergo first pass metabolism?
➤ Aspirin (70%)
➤ Codeine (60%)
➤ Morphine (40%)
➤ Diltiazem (40%)
➤ Propranolol (30%)
➤ Verapamil (20%)
➤ Hydralazine (15–30%)

Reminder of some basic concepts:
➤ An **acid** is a proton (H^+ ion) donor.
➤ A **base** is a proton acceptor (OH^-).
➤ A **weak acid/base** is one which dissociates in water to form an equilibrium with its ions, e.g. $H_2CO_3 \rightleftharpoons H^+ \rightleftharpoons HCO_3^-$.
➤ A **strong acid/base** is one which dissociates readily, but does not form an equilibrium, e.g. $HCl \rightarrow H^+ + Cl^-$.

CHAPTER 5

Drugs and the liver

Why are drugs metabolised by the liver?

Drugs are metabolised to facilitate their excretion. Some drugs are fully ionised at physiological pH and as a result are very polar. These drugs tend to need little, if any, metabolism in order to be excreted by the kidney (*see* Chapter 6 on 'Drugs and the kidney'). Most drugs are more lipophilic and require a degree of metabolism or biomodification in order to be excreted.

The metabolism of drugs in the liver is defined as the modification or degradation of drugs by the liver in order to activate, deactivate, toxify or detoxify drugs in the body.

The majority of metabolic reactions serve to deactivate and aid the excretion of the drugs, often by turning a lipophilic compound to a readily excreted polar one.

The rate at which the drug is metabolised will be an important factor in the intensity and duration of a drugs action.

Some drugs are given as pro-drugs that need to be metabolised in order to become active, e.g. enalapril which must be converted to enalaprilat for its action. Others may have active substrates, such as morphine, or substrates with completely different actions.

How are drugs metabolised by the liver?

The types of reaction that occur can be classified into phase I or phase II reactions. While they may occur in other parts of the body the majority take place in the smooth endoplasmic reticulum of liver.

Phase I reactions:

➤ These normally precede phase II reactions and involve oxidation, reduction or hydrolysis of the drug in order to activate or deactivate it.

➤ The reaction usually adds or unmasks polar bodies in the chemical.

➤ Oxidation and reduction are mainly hepatic, whereas hydrolysis is more widespread throughout the body, e.g. by plasma cholinesterase.

➤ For oxidation reactions the cytochrome P450 system of enzymes is particularly important. These enzymes show genetic variability and their activity can be induced or inhibited by the presence of certain other drugs or chemicals (*see* Table 1.4). This becomes of particular importance when the drugs concerned have a narrow therapeutic window and inhibition of their metabolism will cause toxicity, or induction of their metabolism will render them ineffective.

➤ Drugs undergoing phase 1 reactions include phenothiazines, paracetamol and steroids.

➤ For some drugs, this reaction will be sufficient to allow excretion, but others will require further modification and undergo phase II reactions.

TABLE 1.4 List of common drugs that induce or inhibit the hepatic cytochrome P450 enzyme system

Inhibitors	*Inducers*
Metronidazole	Carbamazepine
Ciprofloxacin	Rifampicin
Fluconazole	Alcohol
Erythromycin	Phenytoin
Ethanol	Griseofulvin
Dextroproxyphene (co-proxamol)	Primidone
Cimetidine	Inhalational agents (enflurane, halothane)
Amiodarone	Smoking
Ketoconazole	Barbiturates
Etomidate	Glucocorticoids
Grapefruit	

Phase II reactions:
➤ These involve adding groups to the drugs and are sometimes referred to as conjugation or synthetic reactions. These groups increase the water solubility of the drugs and allow excretion in the bile or urine. Although they often follow Phase I reactions they may be the only step in the metabolism of drugs.
➤ Phase II reactions include glucuronidation, sulphation, acetylation and methylation.

What drugs can cause damage to the liver?
Drug-induced hepatitis can follow acute or chronic drug exposure. The most commonly encountered drug causing direct hepatocellular damage is ethanol. Chronic alcohol abuse in genetically susceptible individuals can cause progressive inflammatory liver damage, which may result in fatty liver and cirrhosis.

Alcohol damages the liver in several ways:
➤ Ethanol and its metabolite acetaldehyde damage the liver cell and mitochondrial membranes.
➤ Free radicals, superoxides and hydroperoxides generated during ethanol metabolism damage the liver.
➤ Alcoholic hepatitis stimulates the immune system, which generates autoantibodies.

The volatile anaesthetic agent halothane is also known to cause hepatitis, with a mortality rate of 50% in those affected.
➤ Halothane can cause a reversible transaminitis as a result of hepatic hypoxia.
➤ It can cause significant centrilobular liver necrosis in what appears to be an immune-mediated process.
➤ Halothane is oxidised, producing trifluroacetyl metabolites, which bind to liver proteins. In genetically susceptible individuals this causes an autoimmune response and antibodies are generated against the complex.
➤ Risk factors include repeated exposure, female sex, obesity and middle age.

The volatile agents enflurane and isoflurane are also metabolised to acetylated metabolites, but this only involves 2% and 0.2% of the total dose respectively, compared to 20% of halothane.

How does chronic liver disease affect the drugs used in anaesthesia?

➤ Porto-caval shunts occurring in cirrhosis reduce hepatic blood flow and hence the extraction ratio of the drug. This results in an increased drug bioavailability.

➤ Impaired production of albumin results in reduced drug plasma protein binding. This leads to an increase in the free, active component of the drug.

➤ Ascites and the overall increase in total body water leads to an increase in the volume of distribution of drugs.

➤ Reduced metabolic function (phase I and II reactions) leads to prolonged action of hepatically metabolised drugs.

➤ Impaired coagulation (the liver synthesises many of the clotting factors) and liver-induced thrombocytopenia may contraindicate the use of central neuroaxial blocks.

Benzodiazepines:	Metabolism impaired and effects enhanced. These drugs should be avoided.
Opiates:	Metabolism impaired and effects enhanced. Use with caution in reduced doses.
Barbiturates:	Metabolism impaired, though their effects are terminated by redistribution.
Suxamethonium:	Duration of action prolonged as decreased plasma cholinesterases.
Muscle relaxants:	Effects enhanced as usually highly protein bound.
	Hoffmann degradation of atracurium may be reduced in the lower pH associated with severe disease.
Fluid:	Extreme care should be used in administering intravenous fluids as oedema and fluid overload are likely. Also avoid lactate-containing fluids, e.g. Hartmann's as lactate metabolism will be impaired.

CHAPTER 6

Drugs and the kidney

How are drugs excreted from the body?
➤ Most drugs are excreted from the body by a combination of metabolism by the liver and excretion via the kidneys.
➤ Most parent drug molecules and their phase I metabolites are extensively reabsorbed at the level of the kidney tubules, whereas their more water-soluble phase II conjugates are only minimally reabsorbed and readily excreted.
➤ Some parent drugs are almost exclusively excreted by the kidneys without prior detoxification, such that any alteration in kidney function can result in toxicity. Examples include:
  • oxybarbiturates
  • gentamicin
  • furosemide
  • ampicillin
  • sotalol
  • methotrexate.

Describe how drugs are handled as they pass through the kidney, illustrating your answer with examples
The kidney affects drug elimination at three main stages:
➤ glomerular filtration
➤ active proximal tubular secretion
➤ passive distal tubular reabsorption.

Glomerular filtration
➤ The rate of filtration is governed by the glomerular filtration rate.
➤ Drugs that are of low molecular weight (< 60 000 Daltons) and that are not plasma protein bound (PPB) are readily filtered, e.g. fluconazole and ofloxacin.
➤ Most intravenous anaesthetic agents are of low molecular weight but are highly protein bound, e.g. propofol (98% PPB).
➤ Heparin is a large molecule that cannot be filtered.

Active proximal tubular secretion
➤ The rate of tubular secretion is governed by renal blood flow.
➤ It is an energy dependent process and is carrier-mediated.
➤ Two types of carrier exist:
  • those for acidic drugs, e.g. furosemide, penicillin, NSAIDs and glucuronide and sulphate conjugates
  • those for basic drugs, e.g. histamine and dopamine.
➤ Tubular secretion is more important for acidic rather than basic drugs.
➤ Many drugs are actively secreted from the renal blood vessels into the proximal tubules

because most of the renal blood flow (80%) escapes filtration by the glomeruli, e.g. ACE inhibitors and penicillin.
➤ Some drugs compete for the same carriers and limit the other's secretion, e.g. probenecid administered with penicillin and sulphonamides administered with indomethacin.
➤ Tubular secretion can secrete drugs against their concentration gradients. It is an efficient system even for highly protein-bound drugs.

Passive distal tubular reabsorption
➤ As water is reabsorbed along the tubule, the drug's increasing concentration gradient drives the process of passive reabsorption.
➤ Highly lipid-soluble drugs, e.g. fentanyl, are reabsorbed into the circulation as they pass down the distal convoluted tubule.
➤ Some drugs are too lipid-insoluble to undergo reabsorption, e.g. digoxin, aminoglycoside antibiotics and glucuronide and sulphate conjugates from phase II metabolism.
➤ Changes in urine pH can alter the tubular reabsorption of weakly acidic or basic drugs by altering their degree of ionisation and consequently their lipid solubility. This, in turn, affects their speed of elimination.
➤ Weak bases become more ionised (lipid insoluble) in acidic urine and therefore less well reabsorbed.
➤ Weak acids become more ionised in alkaline urine. This is applied clinically in the administration of sodium bicarbonate to alkalinise the urine in overdoses of aspirin and phenobarbital.

CHAPTER 7

Genetic polymorphism

Explain how genetic polymorphism influences drug metabolism. What clinical effects can this have?

This question is a clear lead into a discussion about suxamethonium apnoea, but do not forget about other drugs whose actions are also affected by the recipient's genetics.

Genetic polymorphism is a term that describes the difference in people's genotype and subsequent variation in phenotypic expression of these genes. The enzymes that metabolise drugs are subject to genetic polymorphism, and so there can be differences between individuals in the handling of the same drug.

Suxamethonium:
➤ Suxamethonium is broken down by plasma cholinesterases.
➤ These enzymes are coded for by autosomal genes on chromosome 3. The normal phenotype is Eu (usual). A patient with Eu:Eu will break down suxamethonium rapidly so that its duration of action is around 2–6 minutes.
➤ There are several variations of these genes and deviation from the normal means that the resulting enzyme's activity is decreased. Consequently, it takes longer to break down the suxamethonium and its duration of action is increased.
➤ Abnormal forms of the gene include Ea (atypical), Es (silent) and Ef (fluoride resistant).
➤ The most common abnormality is Ea:Eu. This is carried by 4% of the Caucasian population, and their recovery time following suxamethonium is extended to around 30 minutes. The incidence of this phenotype is higher in Asians and lower in Afro-Caribbeans.
➤ Incidence and prolongation of block:

Ea:Ea	1/3000	≥2 hours
Ef: Ef	1/100 000	≥3 hours
Es:Es	1/250 000	≥3 hours

How would you manage someone with unexpected suxamethonium apnoea?
➤ The problem should be recognised by the lack of muscle contractions in response to supramaximal nerve stimulation applied several minutes after giving an intubating dose of suxamethonium.
➤ If the problem has gone unrecognised during surgery and anaesthesia is turned off at the end of the case, the patient's heart rate and BP might rise as an indicator of awareness in the face of sustained paralysis.
➤ The patient should remain anaesthetised and ventilated until they are able to take good tidal volumes independently.
➤ FFP could be given theoretically to provide normal plasma cholinesterase. However, the risks of giving it cannot be justified in this situation.

➤ The patient and their family should be referred for genetic testing to ascertain their phenotype and the extent of any abnormality.

How is the enzyme abnormality diagnosed?
➤ The diagnosis and extent of the enzyme abnormality can be made using dibucaine.
➤ Dibucaine is a local anaesthetic agent that inhibits normal plasma cholinesterase by approximately 80%, but does not inhibit an abnormal enzyme as effectively.
➤ Benzylcholine is a substrate broken down by plasma cholinesterase.
➤ Benzylcholine is added to the plasma sample being tested and the degree of benzylcholine breakdown is measured. If the plasma of a normal patient has benzylcholine solution added to it, it emits a certain wavelength of light, which can be measured. If dibucaine is added to this solution the reaction is inhibited and so less light is emitted. In patients with an abnormal enzyme, dibucaine does not inhibit the reaction as much and so light continues to be emitted.
➤ The dibucaine number is the percentage inhibition of benzylcholine breakdown by plasma cholinesterase in the presence of dibucaine. A normal number is between 75 and 85, whereas abnormal homozygotes can have numbers as low as 30.

What other drugs are affected by genetic polymorphism?
➤ Mivacurium is also metabolised by plasma cholinesterases and so is subject to the same variations in metabolism as suxamethonium.
➤ The metabolism of codeine to morphine depends on the enzymes CYZ2D6 and 2C19. There are three broad groups of codeine metabolism:
  • Poor metabolisers – get little symptomatic relief from codeine (1–7% of the Caucasian population)
  • Extensive metabolisers – get good relief
  • Ultra-extensive metabolisers – get very good relief and may be at risk of opioid toxicity (1–7% of the Caucasian population).
➤ Alcohol is broken down by alcohol dehydrogenase. The expression of this enzyme varies between sexes and races. Men express more than women and therefore can metabolise alcohol more rapidly. European races express an allele which makes their enzyme more active than that of Asians.

CHAPTER 8

Isomers

What are isomers?
Isomers are molecules that have the same molecular formula but whose atoms are arranged differently. The word comes from the Greek words 'isos' meaning 'equal', and 'meros' meaning 'part'.

How can isomers be classified?
Isomers can be classified as follows:

```
                        ISOMERS
              ┌────────────┴────────────┐
      STRUCTURAL ISOMERS           STEREOISOMERS
    ┌───────┼───────┐          ┌──────────┴──────────┐
  CHAIN  POSITIONAL  FUNCTIONAL  ENANTIOMERS      CIS-TRANS
```

FIGURE 1.5 Classification of isomers

What are structural isomers?
These are compounds that have the same molecular formula but different chemical structure (i.e. their atoms are arranged differently). There are four main forms of structural isomers:
- ➤ chain isomers – carbon skeleton varies but the functional group remains in the same position
- ➤ positional isomers – carbon skeleton remains the same but the functional group varies position
- ➤ functional – carbon skeleton remains the same but the functional group changes
- ➤ tautomers.

Isomers may or may not have similar properties depending on the arrangement of their functional groups, e.g. enflurane and isoflurane.

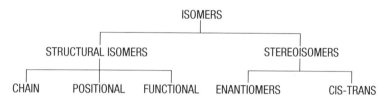

ENFLURANE   ISOFLURANE

FIGURE 1.6 Isomers enflurane and isoflurane

What is tautomerism?
This is a form of dynamic isomerism where two structural isomers (known as tautomers) exist in equilibrium. The position of the equilibrium between the two forms depends on the conditions of the surrounding environment.

> Midazolam, which has a seven-membered ring:
>   • pH < 4.0 – ring open and water soluble
>   • pH > 4.0 – ring closed and lipid-soluble.
> Thiopentone isomers alternate between ketone/enol states.
> Morphine isomers alternate between ketone/enol states.

What are stereoisomers?
These are compounds that have the same molecular formula and chemical structure but different spatial arrangements. There are two main forms of stereoisomers:
> enantiomers and diastereoisomers (optical isomers)
> cis-trans isomers (geometric isomers).

Enantiomers (previously called 'optical isomers'):
> They posses a single chiral centre (usually carbon or nitrogen atom) to which four other atoms are bonded.
> They form the mirror image of each other but cannot be superimposed upon each other.
> They have identical physical and chemical properties.
> They rotate polarised light equally but in opposite directions (they used to be classified as laevo– or dextro– depending on which way they rotated light).
> Each enantiomer is either the R (rectus) or S (sinister) form. This reflects the direction of ascending atomic number of the atoms attached to the chiral centre. (Imagine sticking the 'limb' with the lowest atomic number into the page. Looking down at the molecule, you would now see three groups sticking up. Count from their lowest to the highest atomic number. If the numbers ascend in a clockwise direction the isomer is the R form, if anti-clockwise, it is an S isomer).
> Examples include levobupivacaine and S-bupivacaine, zopiclone and eszopiclone and citalopram and escitalopram.

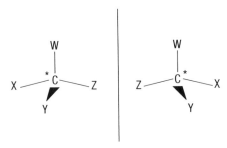

* = chiral centre

FIGURE 1.7 Enantiomers

Interestingly, thalidomide is an enantiomer – one form gives the desired antiemetic effect, but the other is responsible for the teratogenic side-effects. While the drug companies in the 1970s realised this, they did not appreciate that a proportion of the safe enantiomer is converted to the toxic form in vivo, and so marketed it with catastrophic effect. Thalidomide is being used again as a chemotherapy agent.

Diastereoisomers:
> They possess more than one chiral centre and so they cannot form mirror images of each other.

➤ Examples include atracurium which has 4 chiral centres.

Cis-trans isomers (previously called 'geometric isomers'):
➤ They possess a double bond around which the attached atoms cannot rotate.
➤ Cis-form – the groups are arranged on the same side of the double bond.
➤ Trans-form – the groups are arranged on opposite sides of the double bond.
➤ Example includes mivacurium where 36% is cis-trans, 58% trans-trans and 6% cis-cis.
➤ The cis-trans nomenclature only works if the two groups around the double bond are identical.

This is a basic review of isomerism, which is sufficient for the exam. There are many other forms of isomerism, which are not discussed and, as far as we know, have not been examined. For example, there are spin isomers, whose constituent atoms exhibit different spin characteristics and topoisomers, large molecules which may fold and coil in different ways, e.g. DNA.

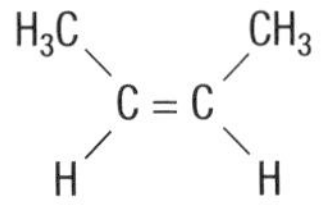

$$H_3C \diagdown \diagup CH_3$$
$$C = C$$
$$H \diagup \diagdown H$$

cis – 2 – butene

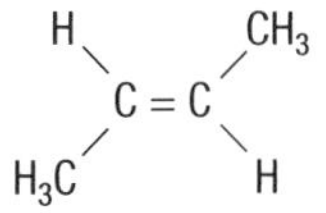

$$H \diagdown \diagup CH_3$$
$$C = C$$
$$H_3C \diagup \diagdown H$$

trans – 2 – butene

FIGURE 1.8 Cis-trans isomers

CHAPTER 9

Exponential functions

Draw a graph showing how the concentration of an intravenously administered drug varies over time

The plasma concentration of an intravenously administered drug decreases exponentially over time, giving a negative exponential decay curve.

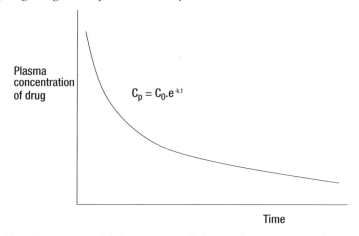

Plasma concentration of drug

$C_p = C_0 . e^{-k.t}$

Time

GRAPH 1.9 Negative exponential decay curve of plasma drug concentration over time

What is an exponential function?

An exponential function describes the situation where the rate of change of quantity of a substance is directly proportional to the quantity of substance at that time. For the graph above this can be equated to:

$$C = dC/dt$$

Where:

C   Drug concentration
dC   Change in drug concentration
dt   Change in time

The formal equation for this negative exponential curve is:

$$C_p = C_0 . e^{-k.t}$$

Where:

C_p Plasma concentration
C_0 Plasma concentration at time zero
e   base of natural log
k   rate constant
t   time

What is 'e'?

e is a mathematical constant and is the base of the natural logarithm. It is sometimes called Euler's number after the Swiss mathematician. Numerically, its value is approximately 2.71828.

What are the properties of an exponential decay curve?

➤ The plasma concentration approaches, but never touches, the x-axis (i.e. it never becomes zero). Instead, it continues to get closer to the x-axis and reaches a steady state known as an asymptote (this takes approximately five half-lives or three time constants – *see* Chapter 12, 'Volume of distribution, clearance and half-life').

➤ The absolute amount of drug that is eliminated per minute varies, but the proportion of drug eliminated per minute is constant, e.g. 50% per hour.

➤ The rate of decline in plasma drug concentration varies according to the plasma concentration of drug present at that time.

➤ The gradient of the curve is the elimination rate constant, k.

Give some examples of exponential processes

➤ **Exponential decay curves:**
  • nitrogen washout during pre-oxygenation
  • lung volumes during passive expiration
  • drug wash-out curves
  • radionuclide materials undergoing radioactive decay.

➤ **Exponential growth curves:**
  • bacterial growth
  • drug wash-in curves
  • lung volumes during positive pressure ventilation (with pressure-controlled ventilation).

Why do we use a log concentration–time curve?

Logging the concentration produces a straight line, which is mathematically much easier to work with than a curve (this graph is actually a semi-logarithmic plot because only the x-axis has been logged because time cannot be logged).

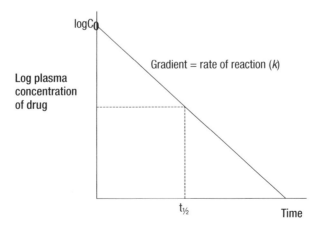

GRAPH 1.10 Log of plasma drug concentration over time

What information can be derived from a log concentration-time curve?

➤ **Elimination rate constant (k)** is the rate of change in plasma concentration per unit time. It is the slope of the line.

➤ **Time constant (τ)** is the time it would take for the plasma concentration to reach zero had the original rate of change continued. It is the reciprocal of the elimination rate constant. It can be read directly from a concentration–time curve.

➤ **Plasma concentration at time zero (C_0)** can be read from the log concentration–time graph (by extrapolating back onto the y-axis – as shown by the dotted line on the graph above).

➤ **Half-life ($t_{1/2}$)** is the time taken for the plasma concentration to be reduced to half its original concentration. It can be read directly from the log concentration–time graph. It is equal to 0.693τ.

➤ **Volume of distribution (V_D)** is the theoretical volume into which a drug must disperse in order to produce the measured plasma concentration.

$$V_D = Dose / C_0$$

➤ **Clearance (Cl)** is the volume of plasma completely cleared of a drug per unit time.

$$Cl = V_D$$

Simple Logarithmic Rules

- Logarithms are a way of expressing numbers as a power of a base.
- The base chosen most commonly is 10.
- So, the logarithm of a number is the power to which 10 would have to be raised to equal that number.

   E.g. log of $100 = 2$ as $10^2 = 100$ (10×10)
        log of $1000 = 3$ as $10^3 = 1000$ ($10 \times 10 \times 10$)

- We also use the 'natural logarithm', whose base is referred to as 'e'.
- $e = 2.718$ (approximately)
- So, the natural logarithm of number X is the power to which e would have to be raised to equal X.

When using logarithms:
- Multiplication becomes addition

   $\log (ab) = \log (a) + \log (b)$

- Division becomes subtraction

   $\log (a/b) = \log (a) - \log (b)$

- Power becomes multiplication

   $\log (a^b) = b.\log(a)$

- Reciprocal becomes negative

   $\log (1/a) = - \log(a)$

CHAPTER 10

Dose–response curves

Draw a dose–response curve for a drug and explain its shape

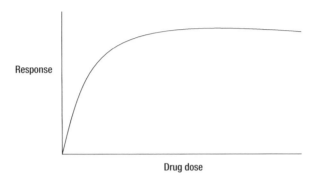

Response

Drug dose

GRAPH 1.11 Dose–response curve

Initially, as the dose of drug increases, more receptors are stimulated, increasing the response. As the dose continues to increase, there are proportionally fewer receptors available for stimulation and therefore the response is proportionally less. Eventually, all the receptors are occupied and so an increase in dose does not effect an increase in response and the graph plateaus.

Why do we log the plot and what shape does this produce?
We log the dose to produce a sigmoid-shaped plot. It is easier and more accurate to extrapolate an estimated response to a given dose using this shape, rather than the unlogged graph. It also allows us to predict the 'effective dose' of the drug, which will produce 50% and 95% of its maximal effect, the ED50 and ED95.

ED50 is the dose of a drug required to produce 50% of its maximal effect, or the dose of a drug that will produce a specified effect in 50% of the sample population.

EC50 is the serum concentration of a drug required to produce 50% of its maximal effect, or the concentration of a drug that will produce a specified effect in 50% of the sample population.

LD50 is the dose of a drug required to produce a lethal effect in 50% of the sample population.

Therapeutic Ratio = LD50/ED50.

Define the terms drug potency, affinity and efficacy
➤ **Potency** describes the dose of drug required to produce a response of a given magnitude. A drug with a high potency requires a smaller dose than one of low potency, to produce the same effect. Usually, the more lipid-soluble a drug, the greater is its potency, e.g. fentanyl (1 µg/kg) is more potent than alfentanil (10 µg/kg).

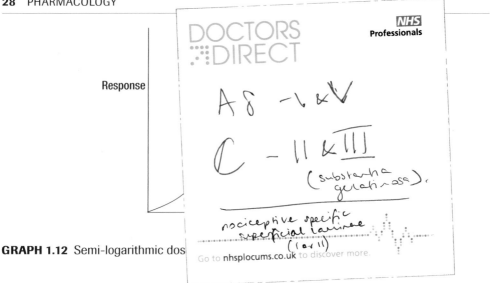

Response

GRAPH 1.12 Semi-logarithmic dos[...]

➤ **Affinity** describes how avidly a drug binds to its receptor. This is irrespective of whether the drug–receptor interaction produces a response or not.
➤ **Efficacy** describes the ability of a drug to produce the maximal response or effect once it is bound to its receptor.

What do the following terms mean?
➤ **Full agonist**
  ● Binds to receptors (has affinity) and produces a maximal response (efficacy = 1).
  ● E.g. morphine acting on MOP receptors.
➤ **Partial agonist**
  ● Binds to receptors (has affinity) but produces a sub-maximal response (efficacy < 1).
  ● E.g. Buprenorphine acting on MOP receptors.
➤ **Inverse agonist**
  ● Bind to receptors (has affinity) but produces the opposite effect to the endogenous agonist (efficacy = –1).
  ● E.g. Flumazenil acting on benzodiazepine binding sites on the $GABA_A$ receptor.
➤ **Antagonist**
  ● Binds to receptors (has affinity) but exerts no effect of its own (efficacy =0). Its presence inhibits the action of agonists of all types, at that receptor.
  ● E.g. Atenolol acting on β adrenoceptors.
➤ **Competitive antagonist**
  ● Binds to receptors at the same site as the agonist and therefore competes with the agonist for this site. This antagonism can be overcome by increasing the concentration of the agonist.
  ● E.g. Vecuronium competing with ACh at nAChR or naloxone competing with morphine at MOP receptors.
➤ **Non-competitive antagonist**
  ● Binds to receptors at a different site from the agonist and so does not prevent the agonist's binding to its receptor site. However, it alters the conformation of the receptor complex and prevents the agonist from eliciting a full response. Its effects are not overcome by increasing the agonist concentration.
  ● E.g. Ketamine acting at NMDA receptor.

➤ **Allosteric modulator**
  • Binds to the receptor at a site separate to that of the endogenous agonist. This alters the shape of the molecule, which either enhances or inhibits the affinity of the agonist for its receptor.
  • Allosteric modulators affect both affinity and efficacy of a drug, as opposed to competitive or non-competitive antagonists, which only alter one of these effects.
  • E.g. Positive modulation: benzodiazepines increase the opening of the chloride channel at the $GABA_A$ receptor, which potentiates the effects of the inhibitory neurotransmitter GABA.
  • E.g. Negative modulation: picrotoxin at the $GABA_A$ receptor.

Draw the log dose–response graph for the following:
➤ **An agonist in the presence of a competitive antagonist.**

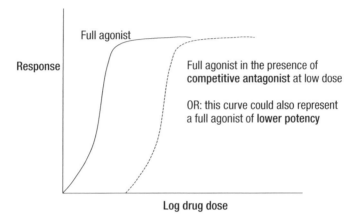

GRAPH 1.13 Semi-logarithmic dose–response curve of an agonist in the presence of a competitive antagonist

➤ **An agonist in the presence of a non-competitive antagonist.**

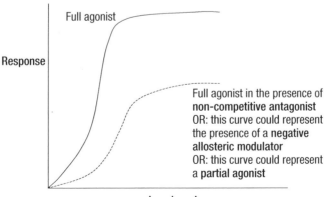

GRAPH 1.14 Semi-logarithmic dose–response curve of an agonist in the presence of a non-competitive antagonist

What is the difference between tachyphylaxis and desensitisation?

➤ **Tachyphylaxis** is the acute reduction in response to a given dose after repeated administration of the drug.

E.g. Ephedrine (an indirectly acting sympathomimetic agent) will display tachyphylaxis due to depletion of presynaptic noradrenaline stores.

➤ **Desensitisation** is the chronic reduction in response to a given dose after repeated administration of the drug. This can be due to structural changes in the receptor and second messenger-dependent systems leading to altered drug affinity and impaired signal transduction processes. Receptor sequestration via endocytosis can also occur, leading to receptor down-regulation and loss of active receptors.

E.g. Dobutamine and adrenaline.

CHAPTER 11

First and zero order kinetics

What are first order kinetics?
- ➤ In first order kinetics a **constant proportion** of the drug is eliminated from the body per unit time, e.g. 50% per hour.
- ➤ The **rate of elimination varies** and is directly proportional to the concentration of drug in the body at that time. This produces an exponential decay curve and is due to **non-saturable enzymes** being involved in drug elimination.
- ➤ The majority of drugs display first order kinetics because the body contains more enzymes than needed to metabolise the clinically effective dose.

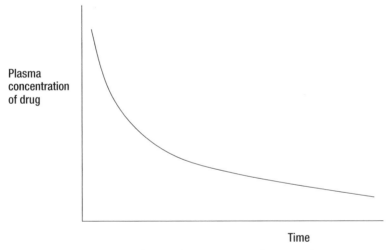

GRAPH 1.15 First order kinetics – plasma drug concentration over time

What are zero order kinetics?
- ➤ In zero order kinetics a **constant amount** of drug is eliminated from the body per unit time, e.g. 10 mg per hour.
- ➤ The **rate of elimination is constant** and changing the quantity of drug available for metabolism does not alter the rate of the reaction. This produces a linear graph because the **enzymes** involved in drug elimination become **saturated**.
- ➤ Ethanol, phenytoin, aspirin, theophyllines and thiopentone display zero order kinetics.

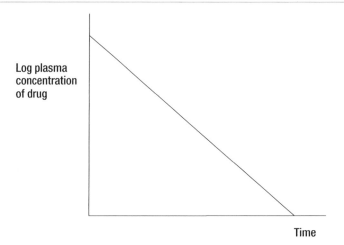

GRAPH 1.16 Zero order kinetics – plasma drug concentration over time

Why is this important clinically?
The therapeutic dose of some drugs is close to the plasma concentration at which the metabolic enzymes become saturated. Once saturated, a small increase in dosing or plasma drug concentration will result in greatly increased availability of the drug.

   If the drug has serious side-effects, these too could become more pronounced. A common example of this is seen with alcohol intoxication, where consuming more than 1 unit/hour will lead to enzyme saturation, and the person concerned will become 'drunk'.

What are Michaelis–Menten kinetics?
These describe the kinetics of the body's enzymes and are used to predict the rate of reaction between an enzyme (E) and substrate (S) to form a product (P).

$$S + E \rightleftharpoons ES \rightleftharpoons P$$

In terms of drug elimination, E represents the enzymes involved in drug metabolism and S represents the plasma concentration of the drug.

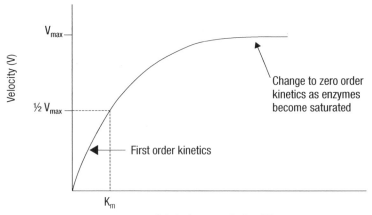

GRAPH 1.17 Michaelis–Menten graph – velocity of reaction (V) over substrate concentration [S]

Michaelis–Menten equation:

$$V = \frac{V_{max} \cdot [S]}{K_m + [S]}$$

V   velocity (or rate) of reaction
V_{max} maximal rate of reaction
[S]   substrate (or drug) concentration
K_m Michaelis constant, which is the substrate concentration at which $V = \frac{1}{2} V_{max}$

➤ At low substrate concentrations: $V \propto [S]$ – it obeys first order kinetics and as the substrate concentration increases so does the rate of the reaction.
➤ At high substrate concentrations: $V \propto V_{max}$ – it obeys zero order kinetics because the enzymes become saturated and the rate of reaction cannot increase any further.

CHAPTER 12

Volume of distribution, clearance and half-life

Define volume of distribution
➤ Volume of distribution (V_D) is the theoretical volume into which a drug must disperse in order to produce the measured plasma concentration.
➤ It cannot be measured directly but instead it is derived from a log concentration–time graph where $V_D = Dose/C_0$ (*see* Chapter 9, 'Exponential function').
➤ Its units are typically mL.

What factors determine the volume of distribution of a drug?
➤ Lipid solubility of the drug.
➤ Percentage plasma protein binding of the drug.
➤ Percentage tissue protein binding of the drug.
➤ Blood flow to the various tissues.

Define clearance
➤ Clearance (Cl) is the volume of plasma completely cleared of a substance per unit time.
➤ It can be derived from a concentration–time graph where $Cl = Dose/AUC$ (AUC = area under curve).
➤ Its units are typically mL/min.

Define half-life
➤ Half-life ($t_{1/2}$) is the time taken for the plasma concentration of a substance to reduce to half its original value (it is equivalent to 0.693τ).
➤ It can be derived from a concentration–time graph.
➤ After five half-lives, elimination is 96.875% complete. Steady state conditions are typically quoted to occur after five half-lives (or three time constants).
➤ Its units are typically minutes (min).

How are V_D, Cl and $t_{1/2}$ interrelated?

$$V_D = t_{1/2} \times Cl \qquad t_{1/2} = V_D/Cl \qquad Cl = V_D/t_{1/2}$$

How can V_D, Cl and $t_{1/2}$ be used to explain the different clinical effects of fentanyl and alfentanil?

➤ Fentanyl is significantly more lipid-soluble than alfentanil (i.e. more potent) and is therefore used in much smaller doses.
➤ Being more lipid-soluble also accounts for the higher V_D of fentanyl because the drug can better penetrate tissues.
➤ The differences in the onset of effect can be explained by the pKa values. Both fentanyl and alfentanil are basic compounds, which means that they become increasingly ionised below their pKa. At physiological pH 7.35 (which is above the pKa of alfentanil) 90% of alfentanil is in the un-ionised form and can therefore penetrate

tissues easily to produce a rapid effect. For fentanyl, physiological pH is below its pKa and therefore the majority of this drug gets ionised such that only 9% remains in the un-ionised form and this explains its longer onset of effect.

➤ The clearance of alfentanil is a lot slower than fentanyl but despite this it has a shorter duration of action because its smaller V_D ensures a shorter $t_{1/2}$.

TABLE 1.18 Pharmacokinetic comparison of fentanyl and alfentanil

Drug	Fentanyl	Alfentanil
Dose (µg/kg)	1	10
Onset (min)	5	1–2
Duration of action (min)	30	10
Lipid solubility	+++	+
pKa	8.4	6.4
Percentage un-ionisied	9	90
V_D (L/kg)	4	0.8
Cl (mL/min)	500–1500	300–500
$t_{1/2}$ (min)	360	120

CHAPTER 13

Compartment models

What is meant by the terms one, two and three-compartment models?
Compartment models are used to design mathematical models that will predict the drug-handling characteristics of the body. They help us calculate the doses and frequency of drug administration and form the basis of anaesthetic infusion regimes used in target-controlled infusions.

One-compartment model
➤ The body is viewed as a single central compartment (C_1) with a defined volume of distribution.
➤ When a drug is administered (rate constant k_{01}) it is assumed to disperse instantaneously and uniformly throughout C_1.
➤ It is also assumed that the drug is then completely cleared from C_1 by elimination alone (rate constant k_{10}).
➤ This model produces a mono-exponential decay curve.

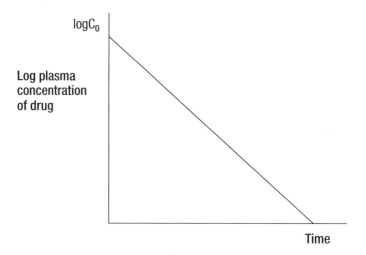

GRAPH 1.19 Semi-logarithmic plot of plasma concentration of drug over time

➤ In reality, this model is far too simplistic because plasma drug concentrations decline due to a multitude of factors including distribution from plasma into different tissues (which can occur at different rates due to differences in tissue perfusion), drug metabolism and excretion. Therefore a less simplistic model with two or three compartments is required.

Two-compartment model
➤ The body is now viewed as a central compartment (C_1 – representing plasma) in conjunction with a peripheral compartment (C_2 – representing tissues).

➤ Additional rate constants apply to this model and plasma drug concentrations now decline due to drug distribution from plasma to tissues (k_{12}) and drug elimination from the central compartment (k_{10}).

➤ This produces a bi-phasic exponential decay curve.

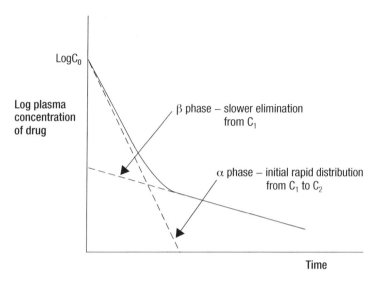

GRAPH 1.20 Semi-logarithmic plot showing bi-exponential decay of plasma concentration of drug over time in a two-compartment model

Three-compartment model

➤ The body is viewed as a central compartment (C_1 – representing plasma), an intermediately well perfused peripheral compartment (C_2 – representing tissues like muscle) and a poorly perfused peripheral compartment (C_3 – representing tissues like fat).

➤ Additional rate constants apply to this model and plasma drug concentrations now decline due to drug distribution into the peripheral compartments of C_2 (k_{12}) and C_3 (k_{13}) and drug elimination from the central compartment (k_{10}).

➤ This produces a tri-phasic exponential decay curve where the distribution part of the curve can be divided into a fast (α) and slow (β) phase followed by an elimination phase.

➤ The distribution to and redistribution from the peripheral compartments along with drug elimination from the central compartment occurs simultaneously and down concentration gradients.

➤ Peripheral compartments can act as stores for the drug, keeping the central compartment full even after drug administration into it has ceased and drug elimination from it continues.

➤ This redistribution of drug into the central explains why the effect of a drug can continue long after its administration has ended and this is an integral concept in target-controlled infusions and context-sensitive half-lives (*see* Chapter 14, 'Total intravenous anaesthesia').

Total intravenous anaesthesia

What is meant by the term 'total intravenous anaesthesia'?
➤ Total intravenous anaesthesia (TIVA) refers to anaesthesia that is provided solely by the intravenous route, e.g. propofol infusion.
➤ It is generally administered as a continuous infusion. This infusion can either be run at a specific rate or titrated to achieve a specific concentration of the agent, either in the plasma (C_p), or at the brain, i.e. the effect site (C_e), by running a 'target controlled' infusion.

What are the indications for using TIVA?
➤ when inhalational agents are not available, e.g. ITU, transfers and field anaesthesia
➤ when administering inhalational agents is difficult, e.g. during bronchoscopy
➤ when inhalational agents are contraindicated, e.g. malignant hyperpyrexia
➤ to reduce post-operative nausea and vomiting
➤ to reduce exposure of staff to inhalational agents
➤ to reduce pollution.

What are the properties of an ideal intravenous anaesthetic agent?
➤ Ideal physical properties:
  • cheap
  • stable and non-reactive with plastics, glass and metal
  • long shelf life
  • water soluble and so easy to formulate and store
  • environmentally safe.
➤ Ideal pharmacokinetic properties:
  • rapid onset and offset, i.e. lipid-soluble
  • minimal accumulation in body tissues, i.e. small V_D
  • rapid metabolism in plasma to inactive products giving a context 'insensitive' half-time
  • no excitation or emergence phenomena
  • no interaction with other drugs.
➤ Ideal pharmacodynamic properties:
  • painless on injection
  • analgesic, muscle-relaxant and antiemetic
  • no effect on patient's physiology
  • no toxic effect
  • no hypersensitivity reactions or histamine release.

What is meant by the term 'target-controlled infusion'?
➤ Target-controlled infusion (TCI) refers to an infusion system where the target concentration of the agent in the plasma or the effect site can be chosen.

What are the pharmacokinetic principles used in designing a TCI?

➤ TCI designs are based on pharmacokinetic mathematical models like the three compartment model (*see* Chapter 13, 'Compartment models').

➤ Pharmacokinetic data sets for the infused drug are incorporated into this mathematical model (e.g. V_D, Cl, $t_{1/2}$, k).

➤ Patient data, e.g. age, weight, height and sex, are also entered into the model.

➤ The mathematical model then predicts the plasma and effect site concentration of the drug and adjusts the infusion rate according to these predictions.

What are the limitations of such a pharmacokinetic mathematical model?

These models are based on several assumptions as follows:

➤ Tissues only have either a high or low blood flow with specific rate constants for distribution, redistribution and clearance.

➤ All people have the same proportion of different tissues.

➤ All people metabolise and eliminate the drug at the same rate.

➤ All people will become anaesthetised at the same target concentration.

There is no in vivo measurement of the actual plasma or effect site concentration of the drug. The data produced are merely predictions based on mathematical models, pharmacokinetic data sets and normograms.

What is context-sensitive half-time?

➤ Context-sensitive half-times (CSHT) are applicable to intravenous infusions of drugs. It is the time taken for the drug concentration to reduce by half once an infusion designed to maintain a constant plasma concentration is stopped.

➤ The term 'context' refers to the duration of drug infusion prior to stopping.

➤ CSHT for a specific drug will vary depending on the duration of the infusion.

What causes context-sensitive half-times?

➤ During an infusion, the plasma will have the highest concentration of the drug in the body and therefore the drug will tend to travel down its concentration gradient into various tissues until tissue and plasma concentrations reach equilibrium.

➤ If the infusion is given for long enough for plasma concentration to reach equilibrium with the tissues, there will be no net movement of the drug between compartments as long as the rate of infusion matches the rate of elimination of the drug.

➤ Tissues with a high perfusion will equilibrate with plasma faster than those with low perfusion. Tissues with a high fat content and poor perfusion will act as a store.

➤ Once a drug infusion has stopped, the drug concentration in the plasma will start to fall as the drug is metabolised and excreted.

➤ The tissues will then have a higher concentration of the drug compared with the plasma and hence drug will redistribute from these tissues into the plasma.

➤ The longer the duration of an infusion, the more drug will accumulate in the tissues, forming a store which can then replenish and maintain the plasma levels as the drug is metabolised and excreted.

➤ This results in the context sensitive half-life.

Which drugs lend themselves well to infusion regimes?

➤ Drugs with a small volume of distribution, rapid metabolism (with no active metabolites), high clearance and short CSHT are ideal for infusions.

➤ Remifentanil, propofol and alfentanil are the three main anaesthetic agents used in TCI.

TABLE 1.21 Context-sensitive half times for various agents

Drug	CSHT after 2-hr infusion	CSHT after 8-hr infusion
Remifentanil	4.5 min	9 min
Propofol	16 min	41 min
Alfentanil	50 min	64 min
Fentanyl	48 min	282 min

Draw a graph showing the context-sensitive half-times of commonly infused drugs

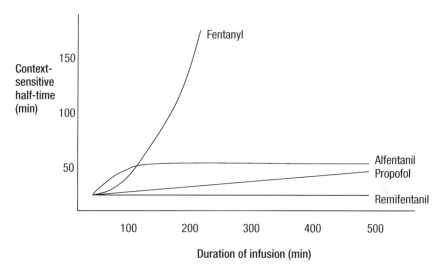

GRAPH 1.22 Comparison of effect of duration of infusion on context-sensitive half-times for various agents

What is unique about remifentanil infusion?
➤ Remifentanil is rapidly broken down by non-specific plasma and tissue esterases.
➤ It has a short elimination half-time ($t_{1/2}$ =1.3 min), high clearance (2.5 L/kg/hr) and small volume of distribution (0.35 L/kg), giving it a relatively constant context-sensitive half-time of 3–10 minutes.
➤ Remifentanil is therefore often said to have a context-'insensitive' half-time.

CHAPTER 15

Induction agents

A complete knowledge of the common induction agents will be expected. This will include the class of drug, mechanism of action (where known), presentation, uses, dose, systemic effects, side-effects, pharmacokinetics and interactions.

The required information for each induction agent is presented in the form of spider diagrams, which allow easy comparison of the drugs. Keep in mind the properties of an ideal induction agent:

Physical properties
➤ Cheap and easy to make
➤ Long shelf life at room temperature
➤ Water-soluble and so easy to store
➤ Painless on injection
➤ Safe if injected intra-arterially
➤ Rapid onset time
➤ Rapid offset time
➤ No excitation or emergence phenomena
➤ No accumulation following infusion
➤ No interaction with other drugs

Biological properties
➤ Analgesic
➤ No effects on patient's physiology, other than rendering them unconscious
➤ No toxic effects

PROPOFOL

USES
- Induction and maintenance of anaesthesia
- Sedation
- Refractory nausea and vomiting
- Status epilepticus

ABSORPTION/ DISTRIBUTION
- Protein binding 98%
- V_D 4 L/kg
- Rapid distribution to tissues
- Rapid elimination ($t_{1/2}$ 1–5 hours, context sensitive) which may be increased following slower release from adipose tissue

MOA
- Uncertain
- May potentiate $GABA_A$ receptor
- May have action at cannabinoid receptor

PROPOFOL (2,6-diisopropylphenol) Phenolic derivative
- 1%/2% white lipid-water emulsion in soya bean oil and purified egg phosphate
- 20/50/100 mL vials and 50 mL pre-filled syringe

DOSE
- 1.5–2.5 mg/kg (adult)
- 2–7 mg/kg (child)
- 4–12 mcg/kg/hr maintenance

METABOLISM AND EXCRETION
- Hepatic metabolism, mainly conjugated to inactive glucuronide
- Renal excretion
- Liver/renal dysfunction has little effect on metabolism
- Clearance exceeds hepatic blood flow, suggestive of extra hepatic metabolism
- No active metabolites

CHEMICAL PROPERTIES
- Poorly water soluble
- Weak organic acid
- pKa = 11 ∴ almost totally un-ionised at pH 7.4
- pH 7.0
- Free radical scavenger
- Physically incompatible with atracurium

EFFECTS
CVS
- ↓BP and SV (15%–25%)
- ↓CO (25%)
- Vasodilatation secondary to NO production
- Bradycardia/ asystole

RS
- Depression
- ↓Laryngeal reflex
- ↑RR ↓V_T
- ↓Response to ↑pCO_2 and ↓pO_2
- Bronchodilation

CNS
- Hypnotic, smooth and rapid induction ↓CPP ↓ICP ↓$CMRO_2$
- Myoclonic movements

GI
- Antiemetic (antagonist at D_2 receptor)

SIDE-EFFECTS
- Pain on injection (improved with new 'Propfol-Lipura®' which has ↑medium chain triglycerides rendering drug more lipid-soluble)
- **Epileptiform movements** (however it is not epileptogenic and is used for treatment of status epileptious)
- Unlicensed in ≤16 yr olds after complications of long-term use in ICU (**fat overload syndrome,** fatty deposits in liver, lung, heart and kidneys/metabolic acidosis/refractory bradycardia)
- **Lipaemia** with long-term use
- **Green urine and hair,** secondary to quinol metabolites
- Increased energy needed for **DCCV**
- Physically incompatible with atracurium

THIOPENTONE

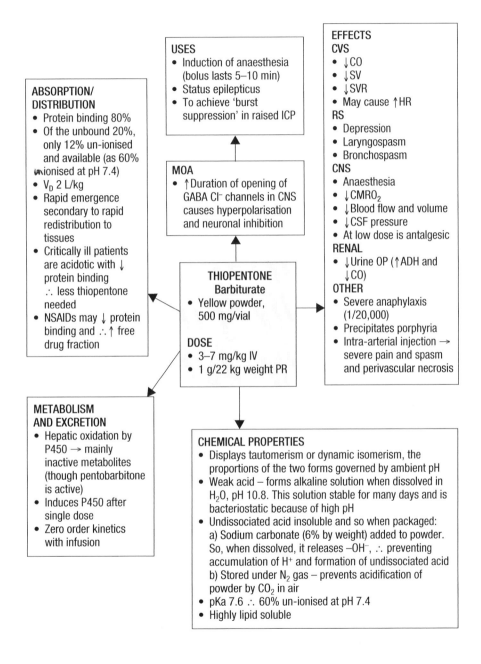

USES
- Induction of anaesthesia (bolus lasts 5–10 min)
- Status epilepticus
- To achieve 'burst suppression' in raised ICP

EFFECTS
CVS
- ↓CO
- ↓SV
- ↓SVR
- May cause ↑HR

RS
- Depression
- Laryngospasm
- Bronchospasm

CNS
- Anaesthesia
- ↓$CMRO_2$
- ↓Blood flow and volume
- ↓CSF pressure
- At low dose is antalgesic

RENAL
- ↓Urine OP (↑ADH and ↓CO)

OTHER
- Severe anaphylaxis (1/20,000)
- Precipitates porphyria
- Intra-arterial injection → severe pain and spasm and perivascular necrosis

ABSORPTION/ DISTRIBUTION
- Protein binding 80%
- Of the unbound 20%, only 12% un-ionised and available (as 60% unionised at pH 7.4)
- V_D 2 L/kg
- Rapid emergence secondary to rapid redistribution to tissues
- Critically ill patients are acidotic with ↓ protein binding ∴ less thiopentone needed
- NSAIDs may ↓ protein binding and ∴ ↑ free drug fraction

MOA
- ↑Duration of opening of GABA Cl⁻ channels in CNS causes hyperpolarisation and neuronal inhibition

THIOPENTONE
Barbiturate
- Yellow powder, 500 mg/vial

DOSE
- 3–7 mg/kg IV
- 1 g/22 kg weight PR

METABOLISM AND EXCRETION
- Hepatic oxidation by P450 → mainly inactive metabolites (though pentobarbitone is active)
- Induces P450 after single dose
- Zero order kinetics with infusion

CHEMICAL PROPERTIES
- Displays tautomerism or dynamic isomerism, the proportions of the two forms governed by ambient pH
- Weak acid – forms alkaline solution when dissolved in H_2O, pH 10.8. This solution stable for many days and is bacteriostatic because of high pH
- Undissociated acid insoluble and so when packaged:
  a) Sodium carbonate (6% by weight) added to powder. So, when dissolved, it releases –OH⁻, ∴ preventing accumulation of H⁺ and formation of undissociated acid
  b) Stored under N_2 gas – prevents acidification of powder by CO_2 in air
- pKa 7.6 ∴ 60% un-ionised at pH 7.4
- Highly lipid soluble

ETOMIDATE

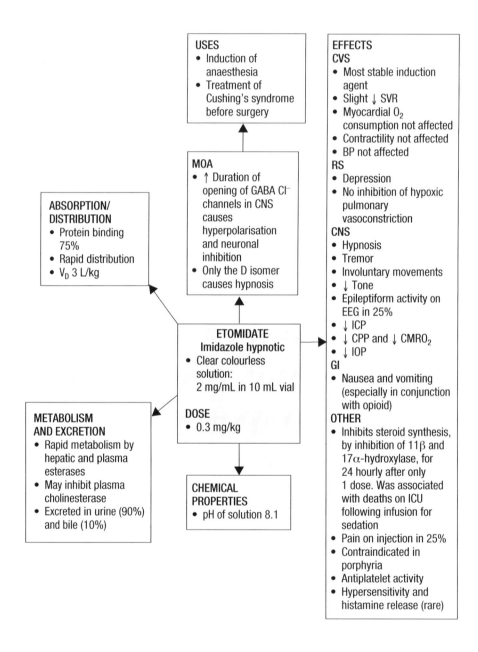

USES
- Induction of anaesthesia
- Treatment of Cushing's syndrome before surgery

MOA
- ↑ Duration of opening of GABA Cl⁻ channels in CNS causes hyperpolarisation and neuronal inhibition
- Only the D isomer causes hypnosis

ABSORPTION/ DISTRIBUTION
- Protein binding 75%
- Rapid distribution
- V_D 3 L/kg

ETOMIDATE
Imidazole hypnotic
- Clear colourless solution: 2 mg/mL in 10 mL vial

DOSE
- 0.3 mg/kg

METABOLISM AND EXCRETION
- Rapid metabolism by hepatic and plasma esterases
- May inhibit plasma cholinesterase
- Excreted in urine (90%) and bile (10%)

CHEMICAL PROPERTIES
- pH of solution 8.1

EFFECTS
CVS
- Most stable induction agent
- Slight ↓ SVR
- Myocardial O_2 consumption not affected
- Contractility not affected
- BP not affected

RS
- Depression
- No inhibition of hypoxic pulmonary vasoconstriction

CNS
- Hypnosis
- Tremor
- Involuntary movements
- ↓ Tone
- Epileptiform activity on EEG in 25%
- ↓ ICP
- ↓ CPP and ↓ $CMRO_2$
- ↓ IOP

GI
- Nausea and vomiting (especially in conjunction with opioid)

OTHER
- Inhibits steroid synthesis, by inhibition of 11β and 17α-hydroxylase, for 24 hourly after only 1 dose. Was associated with deaths on ICU following infusion for sedation
- Pain on injection in 25%
- Contraindicated in porphyria
- Antiplatelet activity
- Hypersensitivity and histamine release (rare)

KETAMINE

USES
- Induction of anaesthesia especially in refractory asthma because of its profound bronchodilator effects
- Sedation on ICU/for short procedures, e.g. dressing change in burns
- Analgesia especially in the military field
- In neuroaxial blockade to prolong its effect
- Drug of abuse

ABSORPTION/ DISTRIBUTION
- Well absorbed orally and IM
- Oral bioavailability 20%
- Protein binding 20–50%
- V_D 3 L/kg
- $t_{1/2}$ 2.5 hours

MOA
- Non-competitive antagonist at NMDA receptor
- Antagonist at MOP receptor, antagonist at KOP and DOP receptors (no interaction with GABA)

EFFECTS
CVS
- ↑ noradrenaline and adrenaline release
- ↑ HR
- ↑ CO
- ↑ BP
- ↑ Cardiac O_2 consumption

RS
- ↑ RR
- No ↓ laryngeal reflex
- Airway maintained
- Profound bronchodilation

CNS
- Dissociative anaesthesia (i.e. strong analgesic and light 'sleep')
- ↑CBF/↑ICP/↑$CMRO_2$ (though new evidence suggests it may be neuro-protective)
- ↑ IOP
- Amnesia
- Emergence phenomena, delirium, hallucinations. Reduced by co-administration of benzodiazepine
- ↑ Muscle tone

GI
- Nauea and vomiting
- Salivation

KETAMINE
Phencyclidine derivative
- Colourless solution in glass vial: 10/50/100 mg/mL
- Available as racemic mix or as S (+) enantiomer (less delirium)
- IV/IM/PO/PR/intrathecal/ epidural administration
- Induction dose: 1–2 mg/kg IV 5–10 mg/kg IM
- Analgesic dose: 0.2–0.5 mg/kg

METABOLISM AND EXCRETION
- Metabolised in liver by P450 to norketamine (30% potency)
- Norketamine metabolised by conjugation to inactive compound
- Excreted in urine

CHEMICAL PROPERTIES
- Water soluble forming acidic solution pH 3.5–5.5

CHAPTER 16

Nitrous oxide

The use of nitrous oxide (N_2O) remains widespread in UK anaesthetic practice despite potential problems, which would almost certainly prevent N_2O being granted a licence if it were discovered today. Examiners will expect a balanced answer illustrating the advantages and disadvantages of N_2O use.

How is nitrous oxide produced?
Ammonium nitrate is heated to 250°C causing it to decompose:

$$NH_4NO_3 \longrightarrow N_2O + 2H_2O$$

If temperature is not controlled carefully during production, contaminants may accumulate in the gas (e.g. NH_3, N_2, NO, NO_2 and HNO_3). Any impurities are removed prior to storage.

How is nitrous oxide stored?
➤ N_2O is stored in cylinders coloured 'French blue'.
➤ It is stored as a liquid, below its critical temperature (36.5°C)

List the physicochemical properties of N_2O
➤ Boiling point –88°C
➤ Critical temperature 36.5°C
➤ Critical pressure 72 bar
➤ Blood:gas partition coefficient 0.47
➤ Oil:gas partition coefficient 1.4
➤ MAC 105% (only under hyperbaric conditions can N_2O produce full anaesthesia)

List its pharmacodynamic properties
Cardiovascular:
➤ Reduces myocardial contractility but increases sympathetic outflow, resulting in a minimal change in blood pressure.
➤ Increases pulmonary vascular resistance and should be avoided in patients with known pulmonary hypertension.

Respiratory:
➤ Causes a reduction in tidal volume and an increase in respiratory rate, resulting in maintenance of minute ventilation.
➤ Blunts the ventilatory responses to both hypoxia and hypercarbia.

Neurological:
➤ Increases cerebral blood flow, cerebral metabolic requirement for oxygen and intracranial pressure.
➤ Effects are more pronounced in patients with loss of cerebral autoregulation, e.g. traumatic brain injury.

How is N_2O used clinically?

General anaesthesia:
➤ As a carrier gas.
➤ To reduce the amount of volatile agent used because of its MAC sparing effect (e.g. 0.5 MAC N_2O + 0.5 MAC sevoflurane = 1 MAC). This is due to its inhibitory action at NMDA (glutamate) receptors and agonist activity at dopamine receptors.
➤ To give faster onset of inhalational anaesthesia using the 'concentration effect' and the 'second gas effect'. N_2O is 30 times more soluble in blood than nitrogen and therefore diffuses more rapidly across the alveolar membrane into the blood than nitrogen can diffuse out into the alveoli. This results in reduced alveolar volume and a rise in alveolar partial pressure and concentration of the remaining gases. This is the 'concentration effect'. Because the concentration gradient between alveoli and blood is now increased, there is faster diffusion of volatile agents into the blood and therefore faster onset of anaesthesia. This is the 'second gas effect'.

Analgesia:
➤ N_2O is a good analgesic, exhibiting agonist activity at opioid receptors and acting at a spinal cord level through modulation of descending noradrenergic pain pathways.
➤ It is mixed with oxygen to form entonox (50% O_2 and 50% N_2O), which is used for pain relief, predominantly during labour.

What are its adverse effects?

Post-operative nausea and vomiting (PONV):
➤ The use of N_2O during general anaesthesia is associated with an increased incidence of PONV. The exact aetiology is unclear but may involve bowel distension, middle ear or opioid effects.

Expansion of nitrogen-containing cavities:
➤ This occurs because N_2O is more soluble than nitrogen and so it diffuses from the blood into air-filled cavities more quickly than nitrogen already in the cavity can diffuse back into the blood.
➤ Use of N_2O results in increased pressure in air-filled spaces, e.g. middle ear, pneumothoraces, endotracheal cuffs (during prolonged surgery) and bowel. It is therefore contraindicated in certain types of surgery.

Bone marrow toxicity and CNS toxicity:
➤ N_2O oxidises the cobalt ion in the vitamin B_{12} complex, impairing its ability to act as a co-factor for the enzyme methionine synthase.
➤ This causes bone marrow suppression and therefore reduced DNA, methionine, thymidine and tetrahydrafolate synthesis. The result is megaloblastic anaemia and subacute degeneration of the spinal cord (dorsal columns) leading to neuropathy.

Teratogenicity:
➤ Has occurred in rats, but never in humans.
➤ The exact mechanism is likely to be multi-factorial, but includes impaired DNA synthesis and α_1-adrenoceptor agonist activity, which is associated with situs inversus.

Environmental pollutant:
➤ N_2O is a greenhouse gas; however, anaesthetic emissions account for a tiny proportion of total nitrous oxide emissions, especially with low flow anaesthesia.

Describe some properties of Entonox
➤ Entonox is the trade name for the mixture 50:50 $N_2O:O_2$
➤ It is stored as a gas in cylinders with a French blue body and blue and white striped shoulders.
➤ A full cylinder has a pressure of 137 bar.
➤ When the N_2O and O_2 dissolve into each other, the resulting gas takes on properties unpredictable from its constituents. This is called the 'Poynting effect'.
➤ The pseudocritical temperature of the mixture is $-7°C$. Below this temperature the N_2O will convert to its liquid phase, in a process called lamination. Anyone using this cylinder will receive only O_2, followed by a mixture of O_2 and N_2O, and finally only the hypoxic N_2O. If the Entonox has been stored below its pseudocritical temperature, the cylinder should be warmed and inverted several times to ensure mixing before use.

CHAPTER 17

Inhalational anaesthetic agents (volatile agents)

Explain the terms 'blood:gas' and 'oil:gas' partition coefficient differences

A partition coefficient is the ratio of the amount of substance in one phase to the amount of it in another at a stated temperature, when the two phases are in equilibrium and of equal volumes and pressures.

At a steady state, the partial pressure of volatile anaesthetic agents within the alveoli (P_A) is in equilibrium with that in the arterial blood (P_A) and subsequently the brain (P_B). As such, P_A gives an indirect measure of P_B.

The blood:gas (B:G) coefficient is a measure of the solubility of a substance in blood and influences anaesthetic onset and offset times.

➤ The more soluble an inhalational agent, the slower its onset and offset times.
➤ This is because its effects on the central nervous system depend on its partial pressure in blood (and subsequently its partial pressure in the brain) and not on the absolute amount dissolved in blood.
➤ Highly soluble agents (halothane and isoflurane) have low partial pressures in blood and more molecules are required to saturate the liquid phase before the P_A can be increased.
➤ As the molecules within the alveoli are readily taken up into the blood, the alveolar concentration and partial pressure remain low, and it takes longer to reach equilibrium (F_A/F_i ratio of 1).
➤ Consequently, the brain partial pressure rises more slowly and the onset of anaesthesia is slower.
➤ Conversely, poorly soluble agents (desflurane and sevoflurane) have alveolar concentrations which rise rapidly towards inspired concentrations, achieving higher partial pressures in alveoli, blood and brain, and onset of anaesthesia is more rapid.

The wash-in curves (F_A/F_i ratio over time) graphically demonstrate the effect of B:G coefficients on onset times for different agents. F_A/F_i represents the ratio of fractional alveolar to fractional inspired concentrations, and different agents achieve an F_A/F_i ratio of 1 (equilibrium) at different rates.

The oil:gas (O:G) coefficient is a measure of lipid solubility and is an indicator of potency. It is inversely related to MAC.

➤ Highly lipid-soluble agents are more potent and a lower MAC is required to achieve central nervous system effects.
➤ The Meyer-Overton hypothesis (*see* p. 53) suggests that when sufficient amount of agent dissolves into a neuronal lipid membrane, anaesthesia is achieved. Using logarithmic scales, MAC can be plotted against O:G for various agents. If this hypothesis were correct, the product of MAC and O:G would be a single constant. In fact, for the older agents, the product equates to 100, whereas for the newer agents, it equals 200, suggesting there may be different sites or mechanisms of action.

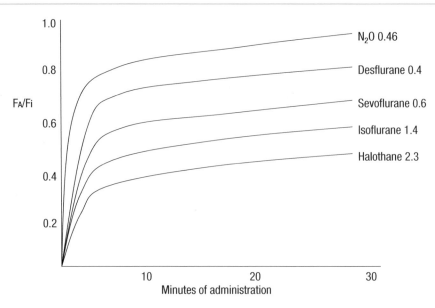

GRAPH 1.23 Wash in curves showing the inspired concentration of inhalational agent (Fi) against alveolar concentration (FA) over time

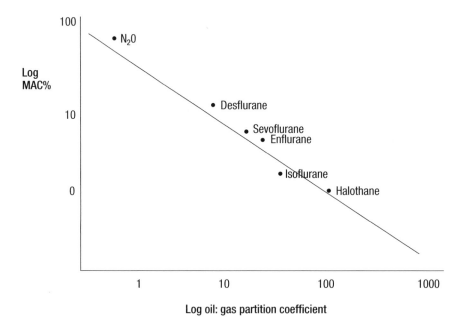

GRAPH 1.24 The relationship between MAC and lipid solubility

Compare the uptake and excretion of isoflurane and sevoflurane

TABLE 1.25 Physicochemical properties of isoflurane compared to sevoflurane

Property	Isoflurane	Sevoflurane
Blood:Gas coefficient	1.4	0.6
Onset/offset	Slower	Faster
Oil:Gas Coefficient	98	53
MAC (in 100% O_2)	1.15	2.05
MAC (in 70% N_2O)	0.56	0.66
Metabolism (%)	0.2	3–5

Isoflurane is more soluble in blood and exerts a lower partial pressure in blood. As it easily diffuses out of the alveoli, it takes longer than sevoflurane to achieve a high alveolar partial pressure. Consequently, its ratio of alveolar concentration to inspired concentration (F_A/F_i) takes longer to approach 1 and its speed of onset of anaesthesia is slower. The converse applies at the end of anaesthesia when the offset time of isoflurane is slower.

Which factors, other than blood:gas coefficient, affect the speed of onset of anaesthesia when using volatiles?

The increase in alveolar partial pressure (P_A) is a balance between the delivery of the drug to the alveolus and the loss from the alveolus to the arterial blood (input minus uptake).

➤ **Inspired concentration (F_i):** If high, there is an increased delivery of drug to the alveolus and a more rapid rise in P_A. In turn, F_i depends on the:
  - concentration set on the vaporiser
  - fresh gas flow rate
  - volume of the breathing circuit
  - amount absorbed by the anaesthetic machine and breathing circuit.
➤ **Alveolar ventilation:** If high, the delivery of volatile agent to the alveolus is increased. In turn, this is influenced by:
  - respiratory depressant effects of the volatile agents with increasing depth of anaesthesia
  - hypocapnia causes a reduced cerebral blood flow and reduced delivery of agent to the brain.
➤ **Functional residual capacity (FRC):** A large FRC will dilute the inspired concentration, resulting in a slower rise in P_A and a slower onset, whereas a small FRC leads to a rapid rise in P_A and a faster onset.
➤ **Cardiac output and pulmonary blood flow:** If high, the agent is taken up from the alveolus more effectively and so the P_A rises more slowly, leading to a slower onset of anaesthesia. A low cardiac output results in a slower uptake into the circulation, achieving a higher P_A more quickly. The onset of anaesthesia is more rapid. The myocardial depressant effects of volatile agents thus have a positive feedback effect on their onset.
➤ **V/Q mismatch and diffusion defects:** These are rarely significant.
➤ **Concentration and second gas effect:** The concentration effect occurs when N_2O is used in high concentration, and refers to the disproportionate rise in alveolar partial pressures of other gases. N_2O is much more soluble than N_2 (35x) and O_2 (20x) and results in a reduced alveolar volume as it diffuses out of the alveoli more rapidly than N_2 can diffuse back in. The reduced alveolar volume results in a rise in alveolar partial pressure and concentration of the remaining gases.

The second gas effect refers to the effect that N_2O has on the speed of onset of anaesthesia of the second gas (volatile). As a consequence of the concentration effect, the volatile agents achieve a rapid rise in P_A, and their F_A/F_I ratio approaches 1 more quickly, leading to a faster onset of action.

The same factors will affect the speed of offset (elimination) of inhalational anaesthetic agents.

How does the structure of an inhalational agent influence its effects?
➤ All volatile agents, except halothane and nitrous oxide, are halogenated ethers.
➤ An ether is a link between two carbon-containing compounds (C-O-C).
➤ Ethers are lipid-soluble but not water-soluble.
➤ A halogen is a member of group VII of the periodic table, which includes fluorine (F), chlorine (Cl) and bromine (Br).
➤ Fluorine is the lightest of the three and lowers the molecular weight (MW) of the compound. A lower MW increases blood solubility, and a higher MW increases potency. Fluorine is the most electronegative halogen and stabilises ethers. It increases the saturated vapour pressure and therefore the compound evaporates less easily (e.g. desflurane).
➤ Halothane is a halogen-substituted alkane (halogenated hydrocarbon).
➤ An alkane is a hydrocarbon with fully saturated bonds, such as methane (CH_4) and ethane (CH_3CH_3).
➤ Alkanes are lipid-soluble and precipitate arrhythmias.
➤ Halogenation reduces flammability.
➤ Halothane is a halogen-substituted alkane (MW = 197).
➤ Isoflurane is a halogenated methyl ethyl ether (MW = 184).
➤ Enflurane is a halogenated methyl ethyl ether (MW = 184). Isoflurane and enflurane are structural isomers.
➤ Desflurane is a fluorinated methyl ethyl ether (MW = 168).
➤ Sevoflurane is a polyfluorinated isopropyl methyl ether (MW = 200).
➤ Nitrous oxide exists in two forms as a hybrid.

What are the harmful effects of inhalational anaesthetic agents?
Inhaled anaesthetic agents undergo metabolism in the liver. The cytochrome P450 system metabolises the carbon-halogen bond to release the halogen ion, which is potentially hepato- and nephrotoxic. The C-F bond is more stable and minimally metabolised, whereas the C-Cl and C-Br bonds are more easily metabolised. Inorganic fluoride ions may be nephrotoxic. Nitrous oxide is only minimally metabolised (0.004%) by gut organisms. Nitrous oxide oxidises the cobalt atom in vitamin B12 complex, which acts as a cofactor for the enzyme methionine synthetase. The resultant bone marrow depression may be apparent by the development of:
➤ subacute degeneration of the spinal cord (dorsal columns) due to inhibition of methionine synthesis
➤ megaloblastic anaemia due to impaired tetrahydrofolate production (important substrate in DNA synthesis).

Sevoflurane administered via a circle system can react with soda and baralyme used to absorb CO_2, resulting in the production of compounds A, B, C, D and E. Only A is potentially toxic (kidneys, brain, liver), but in clinical practice the concentrations produced are much lower than the toxic threshold (200 ppm).

Halothane administration can cause 'halothane hepatitis'. This is thought to manifest in one of two ways:

➤ Reversible transaminitis due to hepatic hypoxia.

➤ Fulminant hepatitis, which is an antigen-antibody reaction. The metabolite trifluoroacetic acid combines with liver proteins (haptens), stimulating the production of antibodies to hapten, and precipitating hepatic necrosis. Risk factors include repeated exposure, female sex, obesity and middle age. Mortality is 50–70%. In theory, it may occur with other agents, but their low rates of metabolism make this less likely.

TABLE 1.26 Metabolic products of commonly used inhalational agents

Agent	% Metabolism	Metabolite
N_2O	<0.01	N_2
Halothane	20	Trifluoroacetic acid, chloride and bromide ions
Enflurane	2	Inorganic and organic fluorides
Isoflurane	0.2	Trifluoroacetic acid fluoride ions
Sevoflurane	3–5	Inorganic and organic fluorides Compounds A, B, C, D, E
Desflurane	0.02	Trifluoroacetic acid

How do inhalational anaesthetic agents exert their effects?

Different hypotheses have been put forward, but no single hypothesis adequately explains their effects.

➤ **Meyer-Overton hypothesis:** This was put forward 100 years ago and describes a link between lipid solubility (oil:gas coefficient) and potency (MAC). The critical volume hypothesis expands on this theory and states that when sufficient amounts of inhalational agents dissolve into the neuronal lipid membrane, ion channels become distorted and synaptic transmission is impaired. The effect of combined inhalational agents is additive.

➤ **Membrane protein receptor hypothesis:** Binding sites for anaesthetic agents on transmembrane proteins have been found. Many ion channels or receptors are likely to be involved including acetylcholine, $GABA_A$, NMDA and voltage gated ion channels.

➤ **Alteration in neurotransmitter availability and action on receptors:** The breakdown of the inhibitory neurotransmitter gamma amino butyric acid (GABA) is inhibited by volatile agents, leading to an accumulation of GABA within the central nervous system and activation of the $GABA_A$ receptor, causing hyperpolarisation of the cell membrane. Volatile agents may inhibit certain calcium channels, preventing the release of neurotransmitters, and may inhibit the glutamate receptor.

➤ **Multi-site hypothesis:** Different inhalational agents alter higher central nervous system function (memory, learning and consciousness) at different concentrations. Furthermore, certain agents, e.g. opiates, may reduce MAC, although this effect is neither predictable nor additive. This implies that there are different sites of action and that inhaled anaesthetics may have both a direct and an indirect effect (via second messengers) on ion channels at various concentrations.

Which neurotransmitters are implicated in the mode of action of inhalational anaesthetic agents?
➤ **Excitatory neurotransmitters**, e.g. glutamate and acetylcholine, are thought to be inhibited.
➤ **Inhibitory neurotransmitters**, e.g. GABA and glycine, are thought to be activated.
➤ Nitrous oxide does not appear to affect the $GABA_A$ receptor, but strongly inhibits the NMDA receptor. It stimulates dopaminergic neurones, mediating the release of endogenous opioids.

What effects do isoflurane, sevoflurane and desflurane have on the cardiovascular system?
All the halogenated agents cause dose-dependent cardiovascular depression with varying effects.

TABLE 1.27 Comparison of the cardiovascular effects of isoflurane, sevoflurane and desflurane

	Isoflurane	Sevoflurane	Desflurane
SVR	↓↓	↓	↓ above 2.2 MAC
MAP	↓	↓	↓
HR	↑↑	↓	↑
CO	↔	↔	↔
Contractility	↔ initially	↔ initially	↔ initially
	↓ at high doses	↓ at high doses	↓ (less than other agents)
Myocardial work and O_2 consumption	↓	↓↓	↓
Dysrhythmogenic	No	No	No
Coronary steal	Yes	Possible	Possible

What is MAC?
➤ MAC is the minimum alveolar concentration, at equilibrium (15 minutes of inhalation), at sea level, in 100% oxygen, at which 50% of the population will fail to respond to a standard noxious stimulus. This is MAC_{50} and is the standard accepted MAC.
➤ MAC_{90} is the concentration required to prevent movement in 90% of subjects.
➤ The stimulus refers to a standard surgical skin incision, and the response refers to purposeful muscular movement.
➤ It is a measure of potency and allows comparison between different agents.
➤ MAC is additive when inhalational agents are administered simultaneously.
➤ MAC awake = 0.3–0.4 MAC, and is the MAC at which eyes open on verbal command during emergence from anaesthesia.
➤ MAC intubation = 1.3 MAC, and is the MAC required to prevent coughing and movement during endotracheal intubation.

Which factors affect MAC?
Factors decreasing MAC
➤ Increasing age
➤ Pregnancy
➤ Hypothermia

➤ Hypothyroidism
➤ Hyponatraemia
➤ Hypotension
➤ Hypoxia
➤ Metabolic acidosis
➤ Acute alcohol
➤ Narcotics
➤ Ketamine
➤ Benzodiazepines
➤ α_2 agonists
➤ Lithium

Factors increasing MAC
➤ Young age (infants and children)
➤ Hyperthermia
➤ Hypernatraemia
➤ Chronic alcohol use
➤ Increased sympathoadrenal stimulation (MAO inhibitors, acute amphetamines, ephedrine, cocaine)

Factors with no influence on MAC
➤ Duration of anaesthesia
➤ Sex
➤ Alkalosis
➤ Hypertension
➤ Anaemia
➤ Magnesium and potassium levels

TABLE 1.28 Summary of the key features of inhalational anaesthetic agents

	Halothane	Isoflurane	Enflurane	Sevoflurane	Desflurane
Chemical	Halogenated hydrocarbon	Halogenated methyl ethyl ether	Halogenated methyl ethyl ether	Polyfluorinated isopropyl methyl ether	Fluorinated methyl ethyl ether
Molecular weight	197	184	184	200	168
Boiling point (°C)	50.2	48.5	56.5	58.5	22.8
SVP at 20°C (kPa)	32.3	33.2	23.3	22.7	89.2
Oil:Gas	224	98	98	53	29
Blood:Gas	2.3	1.4	1.8	0.6	0.4
MAC in 100% O_2	0.75	1.17	1.68	1.9	6.6
MAC in 70% N_2O	0.29	0.56	0.57	0.66	2.5
% Metabolised	20	0.2	2	3–5	0.02
Toxicity	Hepatitis			Compound A	
SVR	↓	↓↓	↓↓	↓	↓ above 2.2 MAC
MAP	↓	↓	↓	↓	↓

(cont.)

	Halothane	Isoflurane	Enflurane	Sevoflurane	Desflurane
HR	↓↓	↑↑	↑	↓	↑
CO	↓	↔	↔	↔	↔
Contractility	↓	↔ initially ↓ at high doses	↓	↔ initially ↓ at high doses	↔initially ↓ (less than other agents)
Sensitise myocardium to catecholamines	Yes ++	No	Yes	No	No
Tidal volume	↓	↓	↓	↓	↓
RR	↓	↔	↑	↑	↑
Bronchodilation	Yes	Yes	Yes	Yes	
Irritant	No	Yes	No	No	Yes++
Response to hypoxia/ hypercarbia	↓	↓	↓	↓	↓
Cerebral blood flow	↑↑	↑(>1 MAC)	↑(>1 MAC)	↑(>1 MAC)	↑
$CMRO_2$	↓	↓	↓	↓	↓
Epileptiform activity	No	No	Yes	No	No
Uterine tone	↓	↓	↓	↓	↓

CHAPTER 18

Neuromuscular blocking drugs

Describe the nicotinic acetylcholine receptor (nAChR)

The nAChR is an integral membrane protein found on the postsynaptic membrane of the neuromuscular junction. It is a ligand-gated ion channel comprised of five subunits: 2α, 2β and 1γ, which are all arranged around a central pore. Its molecular weight is about 250 000 Daltons.

When a molecule of ACh binds to each of the α subunits, the receptor undergoes conformational change, which results in opening of the central pore. This pore is a non-specific ion channel, through with Na^+, K^+ and Ca^{2+} ions can flow, causing miniature end-plate potentials. When the threshold level of depolarisation is reached, voltage gated Na^+ channels open and the action potential is propagated across the muscle.

How does suxamethonium exert its effects?

➤ Suxamethonium is a depolarising neuromuscular blocking drug. Its structure is that of two conjugated acetylcholine molecules and as such, it is much more stable than the natural ligand. Suxamethonium binds to the α subunit of the nAChR and causes the ion channel to open, with resulting muscle depolarisation. This appears as fasciculations as the depolarisation caused by suxamethonium is not orderly.

➤ Suxamethonium is not broken down by acetylcholine esterase and therefore its effects at the receptor are more sustained than the natural ligand. This persistent depolarisation causes the Na^+ channels to become inactive, preventing repolarisation and rendering the end neuromuscular end plate refractory to further stimulation. This produces a flaccid paralysis in the patient. With time, the drug diffuses away from the neuromuscular junction and is broken down by pseudocholinesterase (also known as plasma cholinesterase or butyrylcholinesterase) in the plasma. Now, repolarisation can occur and muscle action potentials are again possible.

What are the characteristics of the ideal neuromuscular blocker?

Physical properties:
➤ Cheap and easy to manufacture
➤ Long shelf life at room temperature
➤ Water soluble and therefore easy to store
➤ Painless on injection
➤ Safe if injected intra-arterially
➤ Ultra rapid onset time
➤ Predictable duration of action
➤ Able to reverse its effects quickly following an intubating dose
➤ No accumulation following infusion
➤ No interaction with other drugs

Biological properties:
➤ Analgesic

➤ No systemic effects other than neuromuscular blockade
➤ No toxic effects

How are non-depolarising neuromuscular blocking drugs classified?
They are classified into two groups according to their chemical composition:
➤ **aminosteroids** – e.g. vecuronium, rocuronium, pancuronium
➤ **benzylisoquinolinium esters** – e.g. atracurium, mivacurium.

How do these drugs work?
➤ Both classes exert their effects by binding to the α subunits of the nAChR and competitively inhibiting ACh.
➤ The drug needs to occupy only one of the α subunits but must occupy at least 70% of all receptors, before any effect is evident.
➤ This feature highlights the margin of safety that exists within an individual. It is well demonstrated in patients with myasthenia gravis where a significant proportion of their nAChR need to be affected before symptoms become evident.

What factors affect the speed of onset of the drug?
Non-depolarising muscle relaxants have bulky structures and are relatively polar. Their volumes of distribution are therefore small and they are not significantly redistributed. They do not undergo first pass metabolism, and are all administered intravenously. Hence, their speed of onset is governed by the concentration gradient between plasma and effect site.

Rocuronium is a much less potent drug than vecuronium, and therefore a higher dose of rocuronium must be given in order to achieve the same degree of muscle relaxation. However, this means that a greater number of rocuronium molecules are being administered which increases the concentration gradient between the plasma and the nAChR. This results in more rapid movement of drug molecules onto the receptors, and therefore a faster onset of action when compared with vecuronium.

What are ED_{50} and ED_{95}?
This is the dose of neuromuscular blocking agent required to produce either a 50% or 95% depression in twitch height. The standard intubating dose is 2 x ED_{95}. When high dose rocuronium is used in order to produce intubating conditions within 60 s, then a dose equivalent to 4 x ED_{95} is used.

What factors affect the speed of recovery from non-depolarising muscle relaxation?
Initial dose:
➤ The greater the dose, the longer recovery takes.

Drug metabolism:
➤ Aminosteroids are minimally metabolised in the liver and excreted in the bile and urine (both as unchanged and changed products). Liver and renal impairment can lead to accumulation of the drugs and therefore prolong their effects.
➤ Atracurium (benzylisoquinolinium ester) is broken down by Hoffman degradation – a process of spontaneous drug breakdown at body pH and temperature. Acidosis and hypothermia will slow this breakdown and prolong the effects.

Drug interactions:
➤ Drugs that induce liver enzymes will reduce the effects of the aminosteroids, e.g. co-administration of phenytoin results in an 80% increase in the necessary dose of aminosteroid.
➤ Co-administration of magnesium sulphate, which competes with calcium, will

prolong the action of neuromuscular blockers by inhibiting the release of ACh from its vesicular stores at the neuromuscular junction. Only 30–50% of the normal dose of relaxant should be used.

➤ Administration of 'reversal agents':
  • Anticholinesterases: Until recently the only drugs available to reverse the effects of non-depolarising neuromuscular blockers were anticholinesterases, e.g. neostigmine, which worked by increasing the concentration of ACh at the neuromuscular junction.
  • Sugammadex: Recently released onto the market and licensed for use with rocuronium and vecuronium. This modified γ-cyclodextrin works by completely enveloping the aminosteroid and terminating its effect as it can no longer interact with the nAChR. The drug–drug compound is then excreted in the urine. Given 3 minutes after an intubating dose of rocuronium, it will terminate its effects in 1.5 minutes.

How does the structure of these drugs govern their effects?

➤ Aminosteroidal drugs are bulky and polar and therefore, they do not easily cross cell membranes and their volume of distribution is low. They contain moieties that resemble ACh which interact with the nAChR.

➤ Atracurium has an oxygen atom in its structure that attracts neighbouring electrons therefore destabilising the bonds between constituent atoms. This leads to breakdown of the molecule known as Hoffman degradation.

PANCURONIUM BROMIDE

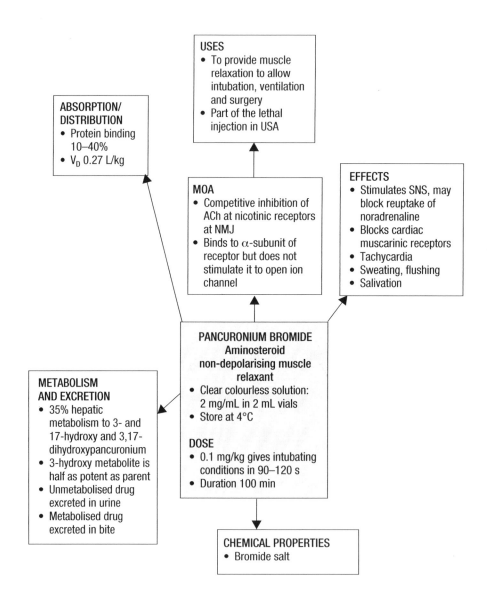

USES
- To provide muscle relaxation to allow intubation, ventilation and surgery
- Part of the lethal injection in USA

ABSORPTION/ DISTRIBUTION
- Protein binding 10–40%
- V_D 0.27 L/kg

MOA
- Competitive inhibition of ACh at nicotinic receptors at NMJ
- Binds to α-subunit of receptor but does not stimulate it to open ion channel

EFFECTS
- Stimulates SNS, may block reuptake of noradrenaline
- Blocks cardiac muscarinic receptors
- Tachycardia
- Sweating, flushing
- Salivation

PANCURONIUM BROMIDE
Aminosteroid
non-depolarising muscle relaxant
- Clear colourless solution: 2 mg/mL in 2 mL vials
- Store at 4°C

DOSE
- 0.1 mg/kg gives intubating conditions in 90–120 s
- Duration 100 min

METABOLISM AND EXCRETION
- 35% hepatic metabolism to 3- and 17-hydroxy and 3,17-dihydroxypancuronium
- 3-hydroxy metabolite is half as potent as parent
- Unmetabolised drug excreted in urine
- Metabolised drug excreted in bite

CHEMICAL PROPERTIES
- Bromide salt

SUXAMETHONIUM

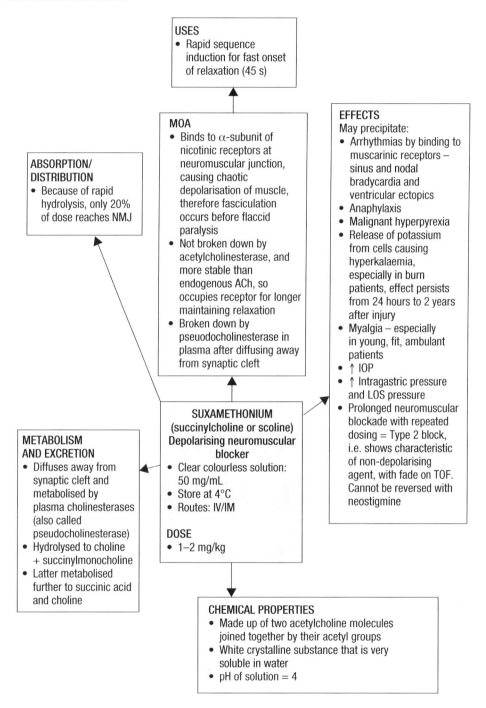

USES
- Rapid sequence induction for fast onset of relaxation (45 s)

MOA
- Binds to α-subunit of nicotinic receptors at neuromuscular junction, causing chaotic depolarisation of muscle, therefore fasciculation occurs before flaccid paralysis
- Not broken down by acetylcholinesterase, and more stable than endogenous ACh, so occupies receptor for longer maintaining relaxation
- Broken down by pseuodocholinesterase in plasma after diffusing away from synaptic cleft

ABSORPTION/ DISTRIBUTION
- Because of rapid hydrolysis, only 20% of dose reaches NMJ

EFFECTS
May precipitate:
- Arrhythmias by binding to muscarinic receptors – sinus and nodal bradycardia and ventricular ectopics
- Anaphylaxis
- Malignant hyperpyrexia
- Release of potassium from cells causing hyperkalaemia, especially in burn patients, effect persists from 24 hours to 2 years after injury
- Myalgia – especially in young, fit, ambulant patients
- ↑ IOP
- ↑ Intragastric pressure and LOS pressure
- Prolonged neuromuscular blockade with repeated dosing = Type 2 block, i.e. shows characteristic of non-depolarising agent, with fade on TOF. Cannot be reversed with neostigmine

METABOLISM AND EXCRETION
- Diffuses away from synaptic cleft and metabolised by plasma cholinesterases (also called pseudocholinesterase)
- Hydrolysed to choline + succinylmonocholine
- Latter metabolised further to succinic acid and choline

SUXAMETHONIUM
(succinylcholine or scoline)
Depolarising neuromuscular blocker
- Clear colourless solution: 50 mg/mL
- Store at 4°C
- Routes: IV/IM

DOSE
- 1–2 mg/kg

CHEMICAL PROPERTIES
- Made up of two acetylcholine molecules joined together by their acetyl groups
- White crystalline substance that is very soluble in water
- pH of solution = 4

ATRACURIUM

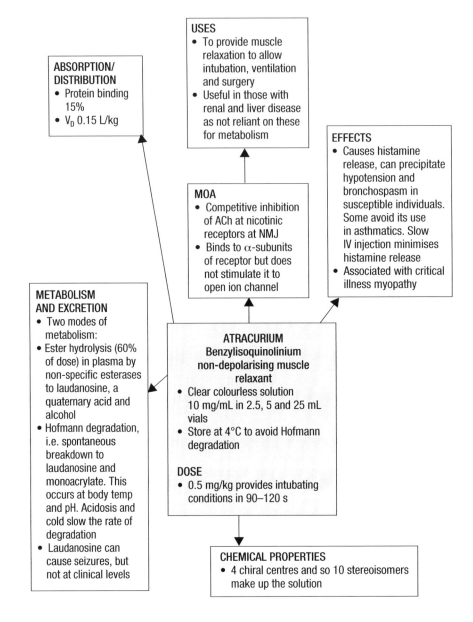

ABSORPTION/ DISTRIBUTION
- Protein binding 15%
- V_D 0.15 L/kg

USES
- To provide muscle relaxation to allow intubation, ventilation and surgery
- Useful in those with renal and liver disease as not reliant on these for metabolism

EFFECTS
- Causes histamine release, can precipitate hypotension and bronchospasm in susceptible individuals. Some avoid its use in asthmatics. Slow IV injection minimises histamine release
- Associated with critical illness myopathy

MOA
- Competitive inhibition of ACh at nicotinic receptors at NMJ
- Binds to α-subunits of receptor but does not stimulate it to open ion channel

METABOLISM AND EXCRETION
- Two modes of metabolism:
- Ester hydrolysis (60% of dose) in plasma by non-specific esterases to laudanosine, a quaternary acid and alcohol
- Hofmann degradation, i.e. spontaneous breakdown to laudanosine and monoacrylate. This occurs at body temp and pH. Acidosis and cold slow the rate of degradation
- Laudanosine can cause seizures, but not at clinical levels

ATRACURIUM
Benzylisoquinolinium non-depolarising muscle relaxant
- Clear colourless solution 10 mg/mL in 2.5, 5 and 25 mL vials
- Store at 4°C to avoid Hofmann degradation

DOSE
- 0.5 mg/kg provides intubating conditions in 90–120 s

CHEMICAL PROPERTIES
- 4 chiral centres and so 10 stereoisomers make up the solution

MIVACURIUM

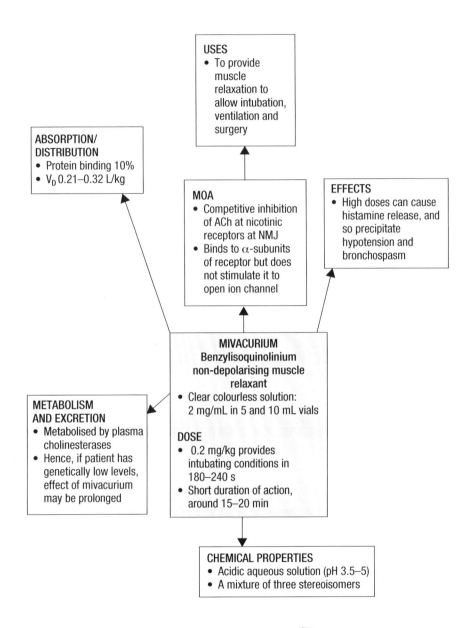

USES
- To provide muscle relaxation to allow intubation, ventilation and surgery

ABSORPTION/ DISTRIBUTION
- Protein binding 10%
- V_D 0.21–0.32 L/kg

MOA
- Competitive inhibition of ACh at nicotinic receptors at NMJ
- Binds to α-subunits of receptor but does not stimulate it to open ion channel

EFFECTS
- High doses can cause histamine release, and so precipitate hypotension and bronchospasm

MIVACURIUM
Benzylisoquinolinium non-depolarising muscle relaxant
- Clear colourless solution: 2 mg/mL in 5 and 10 mL vials

DOSE
- 0.2 mg/kg provides intubating conditions in 180–240 s
- Short duration of action, around 15–20 min

METABOLISM AND EXCRETION
- Metabolised by plasma cholinesterases
- Hence, if patient has genetically low levels, effect of mivacurium may be prolonged

CHEMICAL PROPERTIES
- Acidic aqueous solution (pH 3.5–5)
- A mixture of three stereoisomers

VECURONIUM BROMIDE

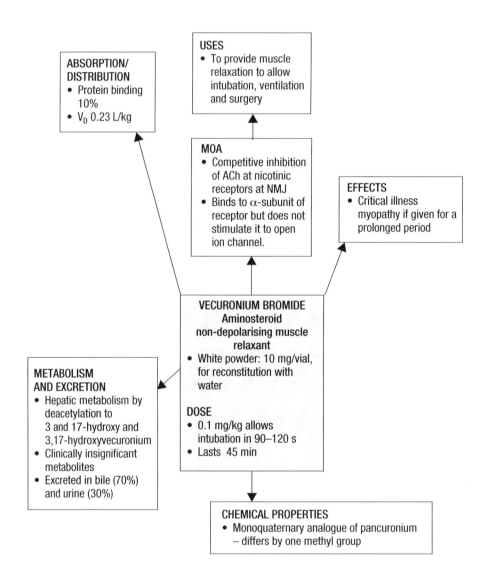

ABSORPTION/ DISTRIBUTION
- Protein binding 10%
- V_D 0.23 L/kg

USES
- To provide muscle relaxation to allow intubation, ventilation and surgery

MOA
- Competitive inhibition of ACh at nicotinic receptors at NMJ
- Binds to α-subunit of receptor but does not stimulate it to open ion channel.

EFFECTS
- Critical illness myopathy if given for a prolonged period

VECURONIUM BROMIDE
Aminosteroid
non-depolarising muscle relaxant
- White powder: 10 mg/vial, for reconstitution with water

DOSE
- 0.1 mg/kg allows intubation in 90–120 s
- Lasts 45 min

METABOLISM AND EXCRETION
- Hepatic metabolism by deacetylation to 3 and 17-hydroxy and 3,17-hydroxyvecuronium
- Clinically insignificant metabolites
- Excreted in bile (70%) and urine (30%)

CHEMICAL PROPERTIES
- Monoquaternary analogue of pancuronium – differs by one methyl group

ROCURONIUM BROMIDE

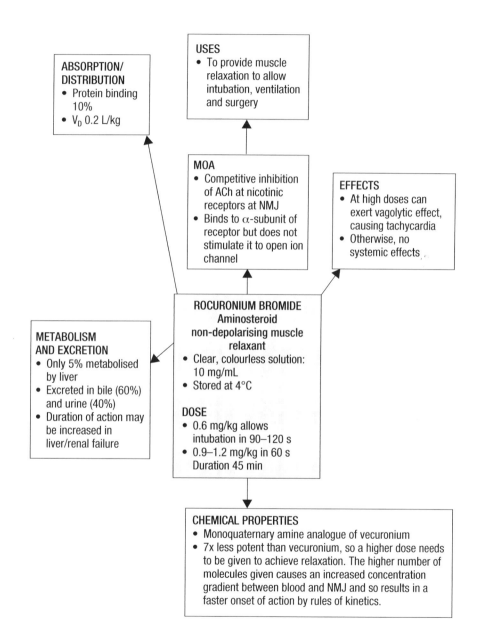

ABSORPTION/ DISTRIBUTION
- Protein binding 10%
- V_D 0.2 L/kg

USES
- To provide muscle relaxation to allow intubation, ventilation and surgery

MOA
- Competitive inhibition of ACh at nicotinic receptors at NMJ
- Binds to α-subunit of receptor but does not stimulate it to open ion channel

EFFECTS
- At high doses can exert vagolytic effect, causing tachycardia
- Otherwise, no systemic effects

METABOLISM AND EXCRETION
- Only 5% metabolised by liver
- Excreted in bile (60%) and urine (40%)
- Duration of action may be increased in liver/renal failure

ROCURONIUM BROMIDE
Aminosteroid
non-depolarising muscle relaxant
- Clear, colourless solution: 10 mg/mL
- Stored at 4°C

DOSE
- 0.6 mg/kg allows intubation in 90–120 s
- 0.9–1.2 mg/kg in 60 s Duration 45 min

CHEMICAL PROPERTIES
- Monoquaternary amine analogue of vecuronium
- 7x less potent than vecuronium, so a higher dose needs to be given to achieve relaxation. The higher number of molecules given causes an increased concentration gradient between blood and NMJ and so results in a faster onset of action by rules of kinetics.

CHAPTER 19

Cholinesterase inhibitors (anticholinesterases)

How do anticholinesterases exert their effects?

➤ They inhibit the action of acetylcholinesterase by occupying its active site, which prevents it from breaking down acetylcholine (ACh).

➤ These agents are used to reverse the effects of non-depolarising neuromuscular blocking drugs, as they increase the amount of ACh available to compete with the muscle relaxant at neuromuscular junction.

➤ They are also used in the diagnosis and treatment of myasthenia gravis and form an active ingredient in pesticides and nerve gases.

How are these drugs classified?

Anticholinesterases are classified according to their duration of action:

Short acting:

➤ Edrophonium (trade name Tensilon)
  - **Duration:** 10–20 minutes.
  - **Mode of action:** Competitive antagonist of ACh at the active site of acetylcholinesterase.
  - **Uses:** In the diagnosis of myasthenia gravis (Tensilon test) – following administration, muscle power improves.

Medium acting:

➤ Neostigmine
  - **Duration:** 1–2 hours.
  - **Mode of action:** Carbamlyates the active site of the enzyme. Once bonded, it is hydrolysed like ACh, but the process takes much longer. It also inhibits the action of plasma pseudocholinesterase and so will prolong the effects of suxamethonium and mivacurium.
  - **Uses:** Reversal of competitive neuromuscular blocking drugs and treatment of constipation on the ICU.

➤ Pyridostigmine
  - **Duration:** 2–3 hours.
  - **Mode of action:** As for neostigmine.
  - **Uses:** Orally, in the treatment of myasthenia gravis.

➤ Physostigmine
  - **Duration:** 0.5–5 hours.
  - **Mode of action:** As for neostigmine.
  - **Uses:** Topical eye drops in the treatment of glaucoma.

Long acting:

➤ Ecothiophate
  - **Duration:** Weeks.

- **Mode of action:** Phosphorylation of the active site of the enzyme. The bond is covalent and the enzyme takes weeks to hydrolyse the drug.
- **Uses:** Treatment of glaucoma.

This class also includes:

➤ Sarin, VX – nerve gases used in chemical warfare.

➤ Tetraethyl pyrophosphate (TEPP) – insecticide.

In toxic doses (e.g. organophosphorus poisoning), anticholinesterases can cause SLUDGE syndrome (salivation, lacrimation, urination, defaecation, gastrointestinal upset, emesis) and cause death by paralysis of the respiratory muscles. Treatment is with antimuscarinic agents, such as atropine and pralidoxime.

What are the side-effects of a conventional dose of neostigmine?

Cardiovascular:

➤ bradycardia

➤ hypotension.

Respiratory:

➤ bronchoconstriction

➤ increased secretions.

Neurological:

➤ miosis and blurred vision

➤ low dose: muscle contraction

➤ high dose: large amounts of ACh at NMJ may render neuromuscular transmission obsolete.

Gastrointestinal:

➤ increased secretions

➤ peristalsis

➤ nausea and vomiting.

Other:

➤ sweating.

To offset these unpleasant effects, neostigmine is usually given with an antimuscarinic agent such as glycopyrrolate.

NEOSTIGMINE

USES
- Reversal of neuromuscular blockade caused by non-depolarising muscle relaxants
- Myasthenia gravis
- Paralytic ileus

MOA
- Binds to esteratic site of acetylcholinesterase (AChE), the enzyme which breaks down acetylcholine (ACh)
- Neostigmine is hydrolysed by AChE, but much more slowly than ACh would be
- As enzymes' active sites are occupied by neostigmine, more ACh is available at the neuromuscular junction (NMJ)
- Increased quantity of ACh at NMJ allows more efficient competition with non-depolarising muscle relaxants

ABSORPTION/ DISTRIBUTION
- Poorly absorbed orally
- Oral bioavailability 1–2%
- Protein binding 10%
- V_D 0.4–1 L/kg
- Max effect in 7–11 min, lasts 4 hours
- $t_{1/2}$ 15–80 min

EFFECTS
CVS
- Bradycardia
- Hypotension

RS
- Bronchoconstriction
- Increased secretions

CNS
- Miosis and blurred vision
- Low dose: muscle contraction
- High dose: large amounts of ACh at NMJ may block neuromuscular transmission as receptors flooded

GI
- Increased secretions
- Peristalsis
- Nausea and vomiting

OTHER
- Sweating

METABOLISM AND EXCRETION
- Metabolised by plasma esterases
- Small amount of hepatic metabolism, these products excreted in bile
- Remainder excreted in urine

NEOSTIGMINE
Anticholinesterase quaternary amine
- Tablets: 15 mg
- Solution: 2.5 mg/mL
- Mixed with glycopyrrolate: 2.5 mg neostigmine + 0.5 mg glycopyrrolate/mL

DOSE
- 0.05 mg/kg IV

CHEMICAL PROPERTIES
- Nil

EDROPHONIUM

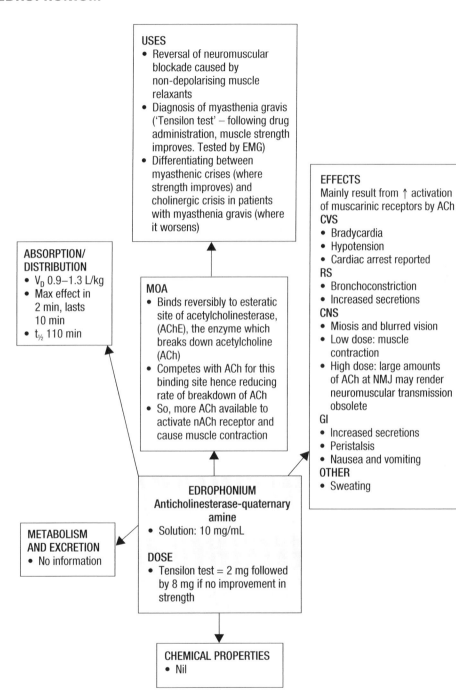

USES
- Reversal of neuromuscular blockade caused by non-depolarising muscle relaxants
- Diagnosis of myasthenia gravis ('Tensilon test' – following drug administration, muscle strength improves. Tested by EMG)
- Differentiating between myasthenic crises (where strength improves) and cholinergic crisis in patients with myasthenia gravis (where it worsens)

ABSORPTION/ DISTRIBUTION
- V_D 0.9–1.3 L/kg
- Max effect in 2 min, lasts 10 min
- $t_{1/2}$ 110 min

MOA
- Binds reversibly to esteratic site of acetylcholinesterase, (AChE), the enzyme which breaks down acetylcholine (ACh)
- Competes with ACh for this binding site hence reducing rate of breakdown of ACh
- So, more ACh available to activate nACh receptor and cause muscle contraction

EFFECTS
Mainly result from ↑ activation of muscarinic receptors by ACh
CVS
- Bradycardia
- Hypotension
- Cardiac arrest reported
RS
- Bronchoconstriction
- Increased secretions
CNS
- Miosis and blurred vision
- Low dose: muscle contraction
- High dose: large amounts of ACh at NMJ may render neuromuscular transmission obsolete
GI
- Increased secretions
- Peristalsis
- Nausea and vomiting
OTHER
- Sweating

METABOLISM AND EXCRETION
- No information

EDROPHONIUM
Anticholinesterase-quaternary amine
- Solution: 10 mg/mL

DOSE
- Tensilon test = 2 mg followed by 8 mg if no improvement in strength

CHEMICAL PROPERTIES
- Nil

SUGAMMADEX

USES
- Reversal of neuromuscular blockade caused by rocuronium and vecuronium
- Can be used confidently to reverse effects, even following an intubating dose of rocuronium

EFFECTS
CVS
- Cardiovascularly stable
- Avoids need to give anticholinesterase and antimuscarinic to reverse neuromuscular blockade, with their attendant side-effects

OTHER
- Also has affinity for pancuronium, though not licensed for its reversal
- Affinity: rocuronium>vecuronium>pancuronium
- Produces rapid reversal because encapsulating the muscle relaxant in the plasma creates a concentration gradient between plasma and NMJ, which causes rocuronium/vecuronium to diffuse away from NMJ into plasma

MOA
- Its ring-like structure enables drug to encapsulate rocuronium and vecuronium in its lipophilic core
- The active site of the muscle relaxant is bound to carboxyl groups in the cyclodextrin so it cannot interact with the acetylcholine receptors at the neuromuscular junction (NMJ)
- Causes reversal of neuromuscular blockade

ABSORPTION/ DISTRIBUTION
- Biologically inactive
- No protein binding
- $t_{1/2}$ 1.8 hours

METABOLISM AND EXCRETION
- Both cyclodextrin and cyclodextrin-aminosteroid complex excreted in urine

SUGAMMADEX
Modified γ-cyclodextrin
Trade name: Bridion
- Approved for use in Europe in July 2008
- Clear colourless solution: 100 mg/mL in 2 mL or 5 mL vials

DOSE
- Moderate block: 2 twitches, 2 mg/kg
- Deep block: 1–2 post-tetanic count, 4 mg/kg
- Immediate reversal from RSI, 16 mg/kg
- At these doses recurrence of blockade is not a clinical problem

CHEMICAL PROPERTIES
- Nil

CHAPTER 20

Antimuscarinic drugs

To answer a question on this subject well, you need to know the structure and function of the autonomic nervous system (ANS). This is covered in a separate chapter (*see Study Guide 1*, Chapter 33). This question could easily go on to explore other drugs which modulate the ANS, such as:

➤ nicotinic AChR antagonists acting at ganglia, e.g. trimetaphan
➤ mAChR agonists, e.g. pilocarpine
➤ adrenoceptor antagonists, e.g. α and β blockers
➤ adrenoceptor agonists, e.g. adrenaline.

How do antimuscarinic drugs work?

➤ Antimuscarinic agents are competitive antagonists of acetylcholine (ACh) at muscarinic acetylcholine receptors (mAChR). These are located in post-ganglionic target tissues innervated by the parasympathetic nervous system (PNS) and also in the sympathetically innervated sweat glands.
➤ These drugs are also called 'parasympatholytic' agents because they reduce the activity of the PNS.

What are the clinical uses of these agents?

Antimuscarinic agents have both anaesthetic and non-anaesthetic uses:

➤ **Premedication**, e.g. hyoscine
  • Used to produce sedation and amnesia.
  • Hyoscine comes in two formulations: hyoscine hydrobromide, which crosses the blood brain barrier (BBB) to produce central effects such as sedation, amnesia and anti-emesis; and hyoscine butylbromide, which does not cross the BBB.
➤ **Bradycardia treatment**, e.g. atropine
➤ **Anti-sialogogue**, e.g. glycopyrrolate.
  • Used prophylactically to reduce excessive secretions in procedures such as fibre-optic intubation.
  • Hyoscine is used in palliative care to reduce excessive secretions (death rattle).
➤ **Bronchodilator**, e.g. ipratropium bromide.
➤ **Antiemetic**, e.g. hyoscine
  • Used to treat motion sickness, post-operative nausea and vomiting and opioid-induced nausea.
➤ **Anti-spasmodic**, e.g. hyoscine
  • Used to treat colicky abdominal pain.
➤ **Co-administered with anticholinesterases**, e.g. glycopyrrolate with neostigmine
  • Used to attenuate the muscarinic effects.
➤ **Anti-parkinsonian drug**, e.g. benztropine, procyclidine and benzhexol
➤ **Mydriatic**, e.g. tropicamide.
➤ **Antidote to organophosphorus and nerve gas poisoning**
  • Troops at risk of chemical warfare carry mini-jets of atropine and obidoxime that can be injected into the thigh.

Can you describe the structure of hyoscine, atropine and glycopyrrolate?
➤ Atropine and hyoscine (also know as scopolamine) are naturally occurring tertiary amines extracted from plants of the deadly nightshade family. They are formed from the esters of tropic acid and tropine or scopine respectively. Being tertiary amines, these agents are able to cross the BBB and can produce central anticholinergic effects.
➤ Glycopyrrolate is a synthetic quaternary amine that cannot readily cross the BBB and so central anticholinergic effects are negligible with this agent.

Compare and contrast hyoscine, atropine and glycopyrrolate

TABLE 1.29 The properties of hyoscine, atropine and glycopyrrolate compared

Property	Hyoscine	Atropine	Glycopyrrolate
Structure	3° amine	3° amine	4° amine
Formulation	Hyoscine hydrobromide (crosses BBB)	Atropine sulphate	Glycopyrrolate bromide
	Hyoscine butylbromide (does not cross BBB)		
Route	PO, IM, IV, TD	PO, IM, IV, tracheal (via ETT)	IM, IV
Adult IV Dose (µg/kg)	5–10	5–20	3–10
Bioavailability	10%	10–25%	5%
% protein binding	11%	50%	Not available
V_D (L/kg)	2	2–4	0.2–0.6
Cl (L/kg)	45	70	0.9
$T_{1/2}$ (hrs)	2.5	2.5	1
Sedation/Amnesia	+++	+	0
Anti-emesis	++	+	0
Anticholinergic syndrome	++	++	0
Mydriasis	+++	+	0
Antisialagogue	+++	+	++
Bronchodilation	+	++	++
Tachycardia	+	+++	++
Placental transfer	++	++	0
Metabolism	+++	+++	Minimal
	Liver esterases	Liver esterases	
Excretion	Urine (tiny fraction unchanged)	Urine (tiny fraction unchanged)	Urine and bile (majority unchanged)

What are the major side-effects of these agents?
The major side-effects produced by these agents result from their antagonistic action on the 'rest and digest' activity of glands, smooth muscle and cardiac muscle. Therefore, their side-effect profile can be worked out logically and classified systematically:
➤ **Neurological:**
  ● 3° amines can cross the BBB and produce an acute central anti-cholinergic

syndrome. The central features of this syndrome include altered mental status, disorientation, hallucinations, agitation, ataxia, somnolence and coma. The peripheral features of this syndrome include dry mouth, mydriasis, blurred vision, paralytic ileus, urinary retention, tachycardia and hot, dry and vasodilated skin.

➤ **Eye:**
  - mydriasis causing photophobia and loss of accommodation (cycloplegia) resulting in blurred vision and diplopia
  - dry eyes (xerophthalmia) due to reduced lacrimal secretion
  - risk of raised intraocular pressure in patients with closed angle glaucoma.

➤ **Respiratory:**
  - Increased anatomical dead space.

➤ **Cardiovascular:**
  - Tachycardia

➤ **Gastrointestinal:**
  - Decreased bowel movement
  - Paralytic ileus
  - Reduced lower oesophageal sphincter pressure – risk of exacerbating reflux in susceptible individuals.

➤ **Genito-urinary:**
  - Reduced urinary tract peristalsis and detrusor muscle tone combined with increased sphincter tone to cause urinary retention.

➤ **Skin:**
  - Impaired sweating results in hot, dry and vasodilated skin.
  - Pyrexia may follow especially in children or in cases of overdose.

ATROPINE

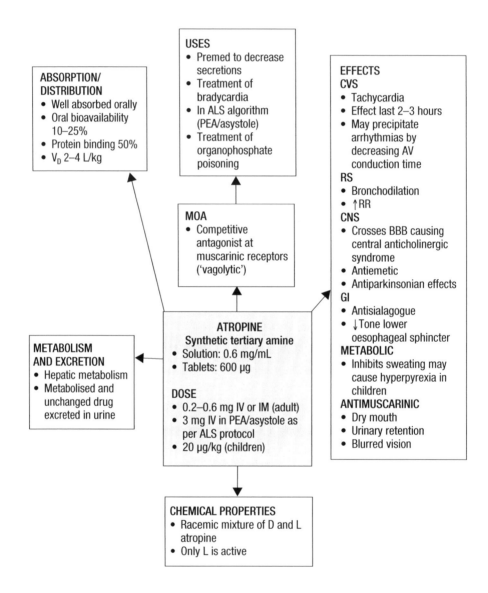

USES
- Premed to decrease secretions
- Treatment of bradycardia
- In ALS algorithm (PEA/asystole)
- Treatment of organophosphate poisoning

ABSORPTION/ DISTRIBUTION
- Well absorbed orally
- Oral bioavailability 10–25%
- Protein binding 50%
- V_D 2–4 L/kg

EFFECTS
CVS
- Tachycardia
- Effect last 2–3 hours
- May precipitate arrhythmias by decreasing AV conduction time

RS
- Bronchodilation
- ↑RR

CNS
- Crosses BBB causing central anticholinergic syndrome
- Antiemetic
- Antiparkinsonian effects

GI
- Antisialagogue
- ↓Tone lower oesophageal sphincter

METABOLIC
- Inhibits sweating may cause hyperpyrexia in children

ANTIMUSCARINIC
- Dry mouth
- Urinary retention
- Blurred vision

MOA
- Competitive antagonist at muscarinic receptors ('vagolytic')

METABOLISM AND EXCRETION
- Hepatic metabolism
- Metabolised and unchanged drug excreted in urine

ATROPINE
Synthetic tertiary amine
- Solution: 0.6 mg/mL
- Tablets: 600 µg

DOSE
- 0.2–0.6 mg IV or IM (adult)
- 3 mg IV in PEA/asystole as per ALS protocol
- 20 µg/kg (children)

CHEMICAL PROPERTIES
- Racemic mixture of D and L atropine
- Only L is active

GLYCOPYRROLATE

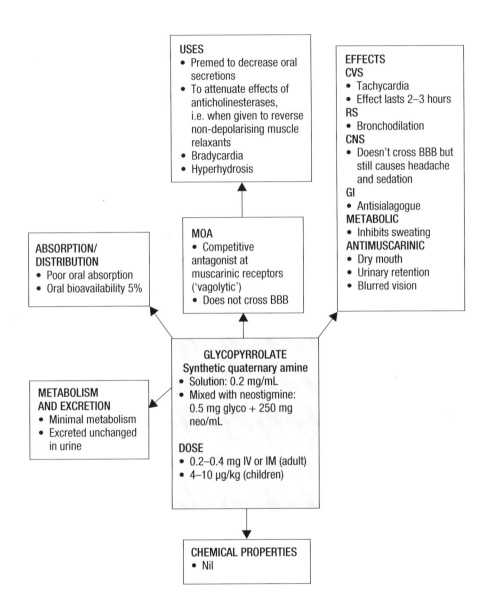

USES
- Premed to decrease oral secretions
- To attenuate effects of anticholinesterases, i.e. when given to reverse non-depolarising muscle relaxants
- Bradycardia
- Hyperhydrosis

EFFECTS
CVS
- Tachycardia
- Effect lasts 2–3 hours
RS
- Bronchodilation
CNS
- Doesn't cross BBB but still causes headache and sedation
GI
- Antisialagogue
METABOLIC
- Inhibits sweating
ANTIMUSCARINIC
- Dry mouth
- Urinary retention
- Blurred vision

MOA
- Competitive antagonist at muscarinic receptors ('vagolytic')
- Does not cross BBB

ABSORPTION/DISTRIBUTION
- Poor oral absorption
- Oral bioavailability 5%

METABOLISM AND EXCRETION
- Minimal metabolism
- Excreted unchanged in urine

GLYCOPYRROLATE
Synthetic quaternary amine
- Solution: 0.2 mg/mL
- Mixed with neostigmine: 0.5 mg glyco + 250 mg neo/mL

DOSE
- 0.2–0.4 mg IV or IM (adult)
- 4–10 µg/kg (children)

CHEMICAL PROPERTIES
- Nil

CHAPTER 21

Opioids

What is the difference between an opiate and an opioid?

The term **opiate** refers to naturally occurring compounds that are derivatives of opium, which have morphine-like properties. Opium comes from the sap of the opium poppy and examples of opiates are morphine and codeine.

An **opioid** is a synthetic substance that stimulates the opioid receptor, e.g. fentanyl and alfentanil.

How do opioids exert their effects?

Opioids work by stimulating presynaptic G_i-protein coupled opioid receptors. Binding of the ligand causes the following events:

➤ closure of voltage-gated Ca^{2+} channels
➤ decreased cAMP production
➤ stimulation of K^+ efflux from the cell
➤ hyperpolarisation of the cell membrane.

This leads to decreased excitability of the cell and therefore decreased neurotransmitter release and pain transmission.

Classify the opioid receptors

There are four main types of opioid receptor, and some of these have subtypes. The receptors were named for the process through which they were discovered:

➤ **μ receptor** (subtypes $μ_1$, $μ_2$, $μ_3$): morphine was used to identify it
➤ **κ receptor** (subtypes $κ_1$, $κ_2$, $κ_3$): ketocyclazocine was used to identify it
➤ **δ receptor** (subtypes $δ_1$, $δ_2$): found in the vas deferens of mice
➤ **NOP receptor**: nociceptin orphanin FQ peptide receptor (most recently identified).

The accepted nomenclature for these receptors is now **MOP** (μ), **KOP** (κ), **DOP** (δ) and **NOP** (N/OFQ), as decided by the International Union of Pharmacology (*see* Table 1.30).

What are the unwanted effects of opioids?

Refer to the spider diagram for morphine (p. 79) for a list of side-effects.

What is tolerance?

Tolerance refers to a decreasing response to repeated dosing of a drug. Over time, a larger dose is needed to produce the same effect. There are two theories as to how this develops: either because of receptor down regulation or because with repeated doses of opioid there is uncoupling of the receptor from its G-protein. Morphine seems to cause uncoupling, but not down regulation of its receptors.

TABLE 1.30 Opioid receptor classification

Receptor Type	Location	Action when Stimulated
MOP	Brain – especially areas involved with sensory and motor perception and integration. Abundant in periaqueductal grey. Spinal cord	μ1 ➤ Analgesia ➤ Physical dependence μ2 ➤ Respiratory depression ➤ Reduced peristalsis ➤ Euphoria ➤ Meiosis
DOP	Brain	➤ Analgesia ➤ Antidepressant ➤ Physical dependence
KOP	Brain Spinal cord	➤ Spinal analgesia ➤ Sedation ➤ Meiosis
NOP	Brain Spinal cord	➤ Anxiety ➤ Depression ➤ Affects learning and memory ➤ Involved in tolerance ➤ Natural ligand may set body's pain threshold, and so administration of an agonist may mean less MOP agonism is needed to achieve pain relief.

What is dependence?

A physically dependent patient will need to repeatedly administer the drug to avoid suffering from withdrawal symptoms.

What is addiction?

Addiction is characterised by the patient's behaviour resulting from their dependence. An addict will:

➤ crave and seek out the drug
➤ have no control over their drug use
➤ use the drug compulsively
➤ continue to use the drug even if it is causing them harm.

What are the symptoms of opioid withdrawal?

Symptoms include:

➤ anxiety and fear
➤ adrenergic hyperactivity
➤ malaise
➤ abdominal cramps
➤ sweating
➤ yawning.

How will you manage post-operative pain control in an opioid-dependent patient?

When treating dependent patients, their baseline pre-existing opioid dosage should be continued and additional pain relief should be administered as required. The patient will be tolerant to opioids and so may need more than the 'average patient' to achieve pain relief. For this reason pethidine should be avoided as large doses may cause the proconvulsant metabolite nor-pethidine to accumulate. It is sensible to include simple analgesia and regional techniques where possible.

If the patient is on a methadone programme, ascertain their daily requirements and continue this dosage perioperatively. If the patient is abstinent, they may be reluctant to use opioids for pain relief, but there is no evidence to suggest that the appropriate use of opioids will precipitate a relapse.

MORPHINE

USES
- Analgesia
- Sedation on ITU
- Palliative care
- CCF

ABSORPTION/ DISTRIBUTION
- Well absorbed orally (from small bowel as ionised in stomach)
- Extensive first-pass metabolism
- Oral bioavailability at 15–20%
- 20–40%PPB
- V_D 3.4–4.7 L/kg
- Low lipid solubility
- Peak effect 10–30 min, duration 3–4 hours

MOA
- Agonist at MOP and KOP G-protein coupled opioid receptors
- Binding of the ligand causes the following events:
- Closure of voltage-gated Ca^{2+} channels
- Decreased cAMP production
- Stimulation of K^+ efflux from the cell
- Hyperpolarisation of the cell membrane and decreased excitability of cell decreasing neurotransmitter release and pain transmission

EFFECTS
CVS
- No direct effects
- If histamine release occurs, may cause hypotension
- Mild bradycardia secondary to ↓ sympathetic tone

RS
- Dose dependent respiratory depression (↓ RR > ↓ V_T)
- ↓ Sensitivity to pCO_2
- Antitussive
- Bronchospasm with histamine release

CNS
- Analgesia
- Sedation
- Euphoria
- Hallucinations
- Meiosis: Edinger-Westphal nucleus
- Seizures and muscular rigidity with high dose

GI
- ↓ Motility
- ↓ Gastric acid, pancreatic and bile secretion
- Nausea and vomiting: CTZ stimulation via 5-HT_3 and dopamine receptors

GU
- ↑ Tone in uterus, bladder detrusor and sphincter muscles – can cause retention

SKIN
- Pruritis
- Rash

ENDO
- ↓ ACTH
- ↓ Gonadotrophic hormones
- ↑ ADH causing hypernatraemia and water secretion

METABOLISM AND EXCRETION
- Hepatic metabolism to:
  - morphine-3-glucuronide (inactive) and
  - morphine-6-glucuronide (active with 13x potency of morphine)
- Excreted in urine
- Neonates have ↑ sensitivity, because of immature hepatic metabolism
- Dose with care in liver impairment

MORPHINE
Naturally occurring opiate
- Tablets: 5/10/30/60/200 mg
- Syrup: 2/10/20 mg/mL
- Suppository: 15/30 mg
- Solution: 10/15/30 mg/mL for IV and neuro-axial use
- **NB** preservative free for neuro-axial use

DOSE
- Oral: 5–40 mg/4 hourly
- Rectal: 15–30 mg/4 hourly
- IV: 0.05–0.1 mg/kg/4 hourly
- IM/SC: 0.1–0.2 mg/kg/4 hourly
- Intrathecal 0.2–1 mg

CHEMICAL PROPERTIES
- Naturally occurring phenanthrene derivative
- Weak base, pKa 8.0 ∴ ionised in stomach

DIAMORPHINE

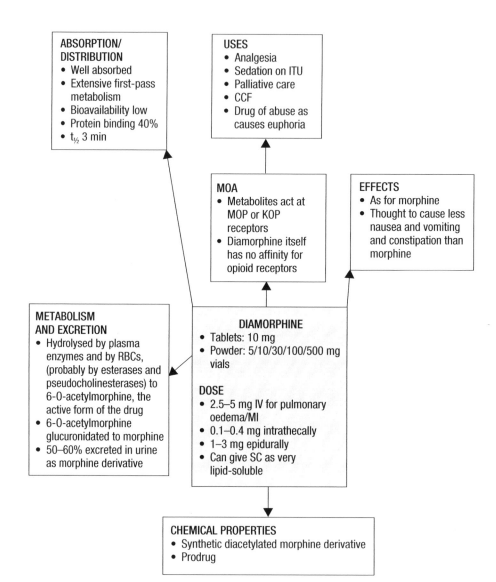

**ABSORPTION/
DISTRIBUTION**
- Well absorbed
- Extensive first-pass
  metabolism
- Bioavailability low
- Protein binding 40%
- $t_{1/2}$ 3 min

USES
- Analgesia
- Sedation on ITU
- Palliative care
- CCF
- Drug of abuse as
  causes euphoria

MOA
- Metabolites act at
  MOP or KOP
  receptors
- Diamorphine itself
  has no affinity for
  opioid receptors

EFFECTS
- As for morphine
- Thought to cause less
  nausea and vomiting
  and constipation than
  morphine

**METABOLISM
AND EXCRETION**
- Hydrolysed by plasma
  enzymes and by RBCs,
  (probably by esterases and
  pseudocholinesterases) to
  6-0-acetylmorphine, the
  active form of the drug
- 6-0-acetylmorphine
  glucuronidated to morphine
- 50–60% excreted in urine
  as morphine derivative

DIAMORPHINE
- Tablets: 10 mg
- Powder: 5/10/30/100/500 mg
  vials

DOSE
- 2.5–5 mg IV for pulmonary
  oedema/MI
- 0.1–0.4 mg intrathecally
- 1–3 mg epidurally
- Can give SC as very
  lipid-soluble

CHEMICAL PROPERTIES
- Synthetic diacetylated morphine derivative
- Prodrug

ALFENTANIL

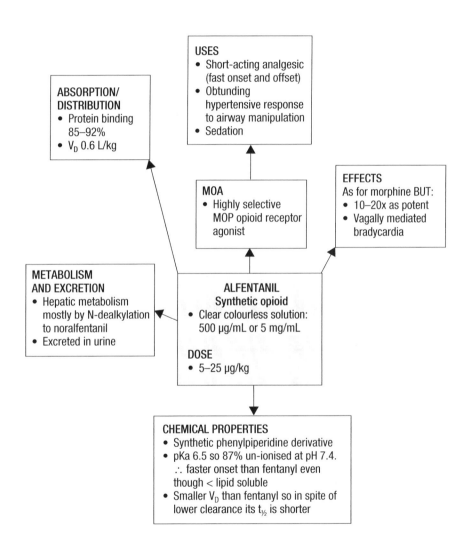

USES
- Short-acting analgesic (fast onset and offset)
- Obtunding hypertensive response to airway manipulation
- Sedation

ABSORPTION/ DISTRIBUTION
- Protein binding 85–92%
- V_D 0.6 L/kg

MOA
- Highly selective MOP opioid receptor agonist

EFFECTS
As for morphine BUT:
- 10–20x as potent
- Vagally mediated bradycardia

METABOLISM AND EXCRETION
- Hepatic metabolism mostly by N-dealkylation to noralfentanil
- Excreted in urine

**ALFENTANIL
Synthetic opioid**
- Clear colourless solution: 500 µg/mL or 5 mg/mL

DOSE
- 5–25 µg/kg

CHEMICAL PROPERTIES
- Synthetic phenylpiperidine derivative
- pKa 6.5 so 87% un-ionised at pH 7.4. ∴ faster onset than fentanyl even though < lipid soluble
- Smaller V_D than fentanyl so in spite of lower clearance its $t_{1/2}$ is shorter

FENTANYL

USES
- Perioperative analgesia
- Obtunds hypertensive response to airway manipulation
- Opioid-based anaesthesia
- Spinal (10–25 μg)/ epidural analgesia (25–100 μg)
- Sedation by infusion
- Chronic pain

ABSORPTION/ DISTRIBUTION
- Absorbed orally, from small intestine
- Bioavailability 33%
- Protein binding 80–95%
- V_D 0.88–4.41 L/kg
- Short duration of action due to redistribution

EFFECTS
As for morphine BUT:
- 50–80x as potent
- Less histamine release
- Decreases stress response to surgery
- Associated with bradycardia
- Chest wall rigidity with high doses

MOA
- Potent agonist at MOP receptor

METABOLISM AND EXCRETION
- Hepatic metabolism
- N-dealkylation to norfentanyl (inactive) then hydroxylation and amide hydrolysis to hydroxypropionyl derivatives
- Inactive metabolites excreted in urine

FENTANYL Synthetic opioid
- Clear colourless solution: 50 μg/mL
- Patches: 25/50/75/100 μg/hr lasting 72 hours
- Lozenges/lollypops: 200 μg–1.6 mg over 15 min
- Patient-controlled transdermal system (PCTS): 40 μg over 10 min

DOSE
- As adjunct during induction of anaesthesia 1–100 μg/kg
- Pain relief, 1 μg/kg, repeat dose titrating to pain

CHEMICAL PROPERTIES
- Synthetic phenylpiperidine
- Highly lipid soluble (600x morphine)
- Highly ionised in stomach (99.9%)
- pKa 8.4 (9% un-ionised at pH 7.4)

REMIFENTANIL

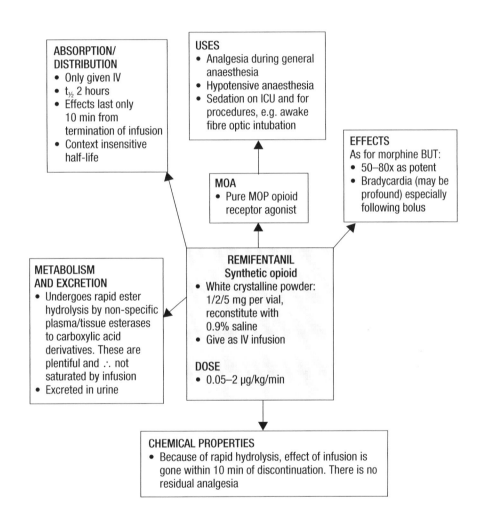

ABSORPTION/ DISTRIBUTION
- Only given IV
- $t_{1/2}$ 2 hours
- Effects last only 10 min from termination of infusion
- Context insensitive half-life

USES
- Analgesia during general anaesthesia
- Hypotensive anaesthesia
- Sedation on ICU and for procedures, e.g. awake fibre optic intubation

EFFECTS
As for morphine BUT:
- 50–80x as potent
- Bradycardia (may be profound) especially following bolus

MOA
- Pure MOP opioid receptor agonist

METABOLISM AND EXCRETION
- Undergoes rapid ester hydrolysis by non-specific plasma/tissue esterases to carboxylic acid derivatives. These are plentiful and ∴ not saturated by infusion
- Excreted in urine

REMIFENTANIL
Synthetic opioid
- White crystalline powder: 1/2/5 mg per vial, reconstitute with 0.9% saline
- Give as IV infusion

DOSE
- 0.05–2 µg/kg/min

CHEMICAL PROPERTIES
- Because of rapid hydrolysis, effect of infusion is gone within 10 min of discontinuation. There is no residual analgesia

PETHIDINE

**ABSORPTION/
DISTRIBUTION**
- Oral bioavailability 50% (subject to first-pass metabolism)
- Protein binding 50–70%
- V_D 4 L/kg
- $t_{1/2}$ 2.4–7 hours
- Crosses placenta where norpethidine accumulates in fetus. Fetal levels peak 4 hourly after maternal dosing. Fetal $t_{1/2}$ 3x that of mother

USES
- Analgesia especially in labour
- Antispasmodic in renal and biliary colic
- Treatment of post-operative shivering

MOA
- Agonist at MOP and KOP opioid receptors
- **NB** not reversed by naloxone

**EFFECTS
CVS**
- Orthostatic hypotension
- Tachycardia secondary to anticholinergic effects

RS
- Respiratory depression
- $\downarrow V_T > \downarrow$ RR
- $\downarrow$ Response to pCO_2 and pO_2

CNS
- 1/10th potency of morphine
- More euphoria
- Less nausea and vomiting
- Miosis and corneal anaesthesia

GI
- Gastric stasis
- Less constipating than morphine

GU
- $\downarrow$ Ureteric tone
- $\uparrow$ Amplitude of contractions of pregnancy

OTHER
- $\uparrow$ ADH
- $\downarrow$ Steroid synthesis
- Severe hypertension with MAOIs
- Norpethide is proconvulsant $\therefore$ caution in high doses

**METABOLISM
AND EXCRETION**
- Hepatic metabolism by N-demethylation to norpethidine (50% as potent as parent) then hydrolysed to pethidinic acid
- Excreted in urine, accumulates in renal failure

**PETHIDINE
Synthetic phenylpiperidine derivative**
- Tablets: 50 mg
- Solution: 10/50 mg/mL

**DOSE
Adult:**
- Oral: 50–150 mg 4 hourly
- IM: 25–150 mg 4 hourly
- IV: 25–100 mg 4 hourly
- Epidural: 25 mg

Child:
- Oral: 0.5–2 mg/kg
- IM: 0.5–2 mg/kg

CHEMICAL PROPERTIES
- Nil

CODEINE

ABSORPTION/
DISTRIBUTION
- Well absorbed
- Oral bioavailability 60–70%
- 7%PPB
- V_D 5.4 L/kg

USES
- Analgesia
- Antitussive
- Treatment of diarrhoea/high output stomas

EFFECTS
CVS
- IV can cause profound hypotension secondary to histamine release $\therefore$ not used via this route

RS
- Antitussive
- Mild depression
- ↓ Response to ↑ pCO_2/ ↓ pO_2

CNS
- 10x less potent than morphine
- Dizziness

GI
- Constipation
- Nausea and vomiting

MOA
- Codeine has low affinity for opioid receptors
- 10% metabolised to morphine – acts via MOP and KOP opioid receptors
- Antitussive effects via specific codeine receptors

METABOLISM
AND EXCRETION
- Hepatic metabolism in three ways:
  1. 10–20% glucuronidation to codeine-6-glucuronidate
  2. 10–20% N-demethylation to norcodeine
  3. 5–15% O-demethylation to **MORPHINE**
- **NB** genetic variability with P450 enzyme CYPZD6 means resulting dose of morphine is variable. 9% UK population and 30% of Chinese are slow metabolisers so codeine will not provide effective analgesia

CODEINE
- Tablets: 15/30/60 mg
- Syrup: 5 mg/mL
- Solution for injection: 60 mg/mL
- Preparations + paracetamol/ibuprofen/aspirin

DOSE
- 30–60 mg 6 hourly (adults)
- 1 mg/kg 6 hourly (children)

CHEMICAL PROPERTIES
- Naturally occurring phenanthene alkaloid – a methylated morphine derivative

TRAMADOL

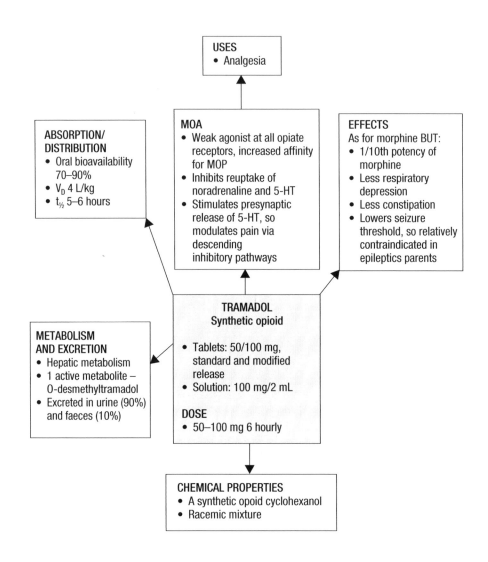

USES
• Analgesia

ABSORPTION/
DISTRIBUTION
• Oral bioavailability
70–90%
• V_D 4 L/kg
• $t_{1/2}$ 5–6 hours

MOA
• Weak agonist at all opiate
receptors, increased affinity
for MOP
• Inhibits reuptake of
noradrenaline and 5-HT
• Stimulates presynaptic
release of 5-HT, so
modulates pain via
descending
inhibitory pathways

EFFECTS
As for morphine BUT:
• 1/10th potency of
morphine
• Less respiratory
depression
• Less constipation
• Lowers seizure
threshold, so relatively
contraindicated in
epileptics parents

METABOLISM
AND EXCRETION
• Hepatic metabolism
• 1 active metabolite –
O-desmethyltramadol
• Excreted in urine (90%)
and faeces (10%)

TRAMADOL
Synthetic opioid

• Tablets: 50/100 mg,
standard and modified
release
• Solution: 100 mg/2 mL

DOSE
• 50–100 mg 6 hourly

CHEMICAL PROPERTIES
• A synthetic opoid cyclohexanol
• Racemic mixture

NALOXONE

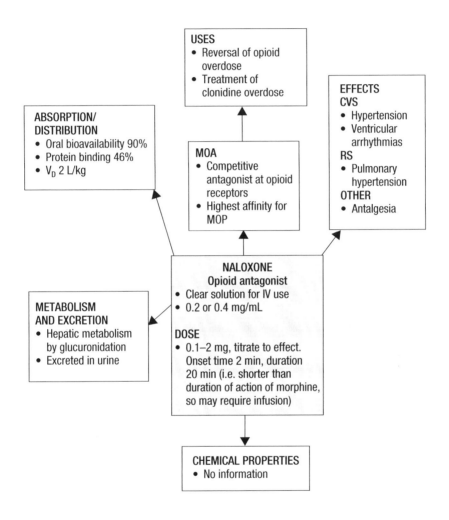

USES
- Reversal of opioid overdose
- Treatment of clonidine overdose

ABSORPTION/ DISTRIBUTION
- Oral bioavailability 90%
- Protein binding 46%
- V_D 2 L/kg

MOA
- Competitive antagonist at opioid receptors
- Highest affinity for MOP

EFFECTS
CVS
- Hypertension
- Ventricular arrhythmias
RS
- Pulmonary hypertension
OTHER
- Antalgesia

NALOXONE
Opioid antagonist
- Clear solution for IV use
- 0.2 or 0.4 mg/mL

DOSE
- 0.1–2 mg, titrate to effect. Onset time 2 min, duration 20 min (i.e. shorter than duration of action of morphine, so may require infusion)

METABOLISM AND EXCRETION
- Hepatic metabolism by glucuronidation
- Excreted in urine

CHEMICAL PROPERTIES
- No information

CHAPTER 22

Local anaesthetics

Local anaesthetic drugs are extensively used by anaesthetists in everyday clinical practice and therefore their pharmacology makes a good SOE question incorporating both basic pharmacology and neuronal physiology.

How are local anaesthetics classified?

All local anaesthetics are composed of an aromatic group linked to an amine group via an intermediate link chain. It is the nature of this link which classifies local anaesthetics as either esters or amides.

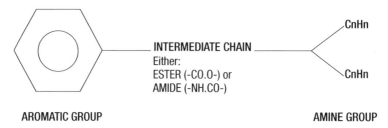

FIGURE 1.31 Schematic representation of the structures of local anaesthetics

Amide local anaesthetics

➤ The amides all contain an 'i' in the drug name followed by 'caine', e.g. lign*o*caine, bupiva*caine*, levobupiva*caine*, ropiva*caine*, prilo*caine* and etido*caine*.
➤ Amides are extensively bound to α_1-acid glycoprotein and albumin in the plasma. Binding decreases with a reduction in pH, so that hypoxia and acidosis can lead to toxicity.
➤ Amides undergo hepatic metabolism by hepatic amidases. Therefore, metabolism is affected in conditions resulting in reduced hepatic blood flow.
➤ Local anaesthetic preparations may contain the preservative sodium metabisulphite or methyl parahydroxybenzoate. These preparations should not be used for subarachnoid injection, as they have been associated with arachnoiditis.
➤ Amides are stable in solution and have a shelf life of approximately 2 years.

Ester local anaesthetics

➤ Examples of esters include cocaine, amethocaine and procaine.
    (A way to remember: **CAPE:** Cocaine, Amethocaine, Procaine = Esters)
➤ Esters undergo hydrolysis by pseudocholinesterases found principally in plasma.
➤ Compared to amides, esters are unstable in solution, and the incidence of hypersensitivity reactions is greater with esters, often due to the breakdown product p-aminobenzoic acid (PABA).

How do local anaesthetics exert their effects?
➤ Local anaesthetics act by blocking sodium channels.
➤ They are weak bases with a pKa > 7.4. This means that they are ionised at physiological pH (7.4).
➤ Open sodium channel block – In the un-ionised form the local anaesthetics are lipid-soluble, which allows transfer of the drug across the neuronal membrane into the axoplasm (pH 7.1), where the drug subsequently becomes ionised, blocking the sodium channels in the neuronal membrane from 'inside'. This stabilises the membrane and prevents the generation of further action potentials. Local anaesthetics bind more avidly to sodium channels which are inactivated or open, and so they are more likely to affect nerves that have a rapid firing rate. Pain and sensation nerves fire at a higher frequency than motor and so they are blocked preferentially, though all excitable membranes can be affected. This is called 'state dependent blockade'.
➤ Closed sodium channel block (membrane expansion theory) – The un-ionised local anaesthetic dissolves in the neuronal membrane resulting in swelling of the neuronal membrane and consequent physical inactivation of neuronal sodium channels preventing depolarisation of the neuron.

What factors govern the potency of a local anaesthetic?
➤ The more lipid-soluble the drug, the greater its potency, e.g. bupivacaine is seven times more lipid-soluble than lignocaine and therefore more potent.

What factors govern the duration of action?
➤ The more protein-bound the drug, the longer its duration of action, e.g. bupivacaine is 95% protein-bound and has a longer duration of action than lignocaine, which is 65% protein-bound.
➤ Addition of vasoconstrictors, such as adrenaline, also prolongs the duration of action by reducing washout of the drug into the bloodstream.

What factors govern the speed of onset?
➤ Speed of onset of action is closely related to the pKa and the resulting degree of ionisation.
➤ Local anaesthetics with a lower pKa (close to pH 7.4) will have a higher un-ionised fraction than those with a higher pKa. This means that a greater proportion of the administered dose will be available to cross the neuronal membrane, and so the drug will take effect more quickly.
  • At physiological pH (7.4), bupivacaine (pKa 8.1) is 15% un-ionised. Lignocaine (pKa 7.9) is 25% un-ionised and therefore has a faster onset of action.
➤ Clinically, bicarbonate may be added to some epidural solutions to raise the pH of the solution and therefore cause the local anaesthetic to be more un-ionised, resulting in faster onset of block.
➤ Infected tissue and abscesses are associated with a reduced local pH. This results in a higher fraction of the local anaesthetic becoming ionised, reducing its efficacy. Reducing efficacy further, is the increased local blood flow to the infected area, causing local anaesthetic washout.

How does the rate of systemic vascular absorption of local anaesthetic agents vary?
The site of injection is important especially in terms of toxicity as the rate of systemic vascular absorption of local anaesthetic varies:
➤ Intercostal space > Caudal > Epidural > Brachial Plexus > Femoral > Subcutaneous

What are the salient features of the commonly used local anaesthetics?

Lignocaine:
➤ Amide.
➤ Fast onset (pKa 7.9).
➤ Medium duration of action (70% protein bound).
➤ Moderate vasodilatation.
➤ Max dose 3 mg/kg or 7 mg/kg with adrenaline.

Bupivacaine:
➤ Amide.
➤ Racemic mixture of R and S enantiomers.
➤ Long duration of action (95% protein bound).
➤ Max dose 2 mg/kg.
➤ Extremely cardiotoxic in overdose.

Levobupivacaine
➤ Amide.
➤ S enantiomer of bupivacaine.
➤ Long duration of action (95% protein bound).
➤ Less cardiotoxic in overdose than bupivacaine.
➤ Max dose 2 mg/kg.

Ropivacaine:
➤ Amide.
➤ Long duration of action (94% protein bound).
➤ More selective sensory neuronal blockade, less motor block.
➤ Less cardiotoxic than both bupivacaine and levobupivacaine.
➤ Max dose 3.5 mg/kg.

Cocaine:
➤ Ester.
➤ Short duration of action.
➤ Profound vasoconstriction – constituent of Moffat's solution (topical).
➤ Blocks neuronal reuptake 1 and stimulates CNS.
➤ Side-effects include hypertension, hallucinations, seizures and coronary ischaemia.
➤ Max dose 3 mg/kg.

CHAPTER 23

Antiemetics and prokinetics

The physiology of nausea and vomiting is covered in *Study Guide 1*, Chapter 20.

Which receptors play a role in the stimulation of vomiting?
The chemoreceptor trigger zone (CTZ) lies close to the area postrema on the floor of the fourth ventricle, outside the blood brain barrier. It is well placed to detect blood-borne toxins. It has many receptors including:
➤ histamine (H_1)
➤ muscarinic (mAChR)
➤ dopaminergic (D_2)
➤ serotonergic ($5-HT_3$)
➤ opioid
➤ α_1 and α_2 adrenoceptors.

The CTZ communicates with the vomiting centre located within the medulla. This centre also possesses receptors including:
➤ dopaminergic
➤ muscarinic
➤ serotonergic.

Stimulation of these receptors may ultimately lead to the activation of the vomiting centre and therefore these receptors are targeted by the use of antiemetic drugs.

Give examples of drugs that act at each site
➤ **Histamine receptors** (e.g. cyclizine and cinnarizine):
  ● Antihistamines exert their antiemetic action at H_1 receptors within the CNS. The sedative side-effect of these drugs may also contribute to their efficacy.
  ● Antihistamines are useful in the treatment of motion sickness, post-operative nausea and vomiting (PONV) and vestibular disorders causing vertigo.
  ● Side-effects include dry mouth, urinary retention, blurred vision and sedation. Cyclizine causes tachycardia if given intravenously, and more rarely can cause extrapyramidal effects and confusion.
➤ **Muscarinic receptors** (e.g. atropine and hyoscine)
  ● The antimuscarinic (or anticholinergic) drugs act on muscarinic receptors at the vomiting centre and also in the gastrointestinal tract (GIT). Here, they are antispasmodic and decrease salivary and gastric secretions, consequently reducing gastric distension.
  ● They are the most effective therapy available for motion sickness, and are also effective for opioid-induced nausea.
  ● Side-effects are predictable, and include dry mouth, blurred vision, urinary retention, tachycardia and sedation.
➤ **Dopaminergic receptors** (e.g. phenothiazines, metoclopramide, domperidone and butyrophenones)

- Phenothiazines (e.g. prochlorperazine, chlorpromazine and promethazine) act on both the dopaminergic receptors at the CTZ and the muscarinic receptors at the vomiting centre.
- Prochlorperazine's (Stemetil) side-effects include extrapyramidal symptoms, especially in children.
- Chlorpromazine is mainly used in the terminally ill as its use is limited by its serious side-effects which include extrapyramidal symptoms, sedation, impaired temperature regulation, increased growth hormone and prolactin release, agranulocytosis, haemolytic anaemia and leucopenia.
- Promethazine is also an antihistamine. It causes profound sedation, which often precludes its use as an antiemetic.
- Metoclopramide is a dopamine antagonist at the CTZ but also works directly on the GIT causing increased gastric motility. It is an effective antiemetic in gastrointestinal and biliary disorders. Its side-effects include acute dystonic reactions (particularly oculogyric crises in young women and the very elderly), sedation, diarrhoea and neuroleptic malignant syndrome.
- Domperidone is a dopamine antagonist at the CTZ. It is of particular use in the treatment of nausea and vomiting associated with cytotoxic therapy. It does not cross the blood brain barrier and so is relatively free of side-effects. It can rarely cause GIT disturbances and hyperprolactinaemia.
- Butyrophenones (e.g. droperidol, benperidol and haloperidol) are dopamine antagonists at the CTZ. They are also mild histamine antagonists and anticholinergics. They have many side-effects including extrapyramidal symptoms, neuroleptic malignant syndrome, altered temperature regulation, hypotension, tachycardia, arrhythmias and endocrine effects including weight gain and galactorrhoea.
- Droperidol is an effective antiemetic but it causes dissociation and dysphoria, which limit its use.
- Benperidol and haloperidol are prescribed for their anti-psychotic actions, and are not used to treat nausea.
➤ **5-HT$_3$ receptors** (e.g. ondansetron and granisetron)
  - There are four types of serotonergic receptors but 5-HT$_3$ receptors are abundant at the CTZ, and are also found in the GIT.
  - The 5-HT$_3$ receptor antagonists are effective in the treatment and prevention of PONV and the nausea and vomiting associated with chemotherapy.
  - Side-effects include headache, flushing, diarrhoea, constipation, drowsiness, tachycardia, bradycardia and ECG changes.
➤ **Steroids** (e.g. dexamethasone and methylprednisolone)
  - High doses of dexamethasone and methylprednisolone are effective in the treatment of nausea caused by cytotoxic agents and in PONV. Dexamethasone may be used alone or in combination for the prevention and treatment of PONV, but its mode of action is unknown.

Which drugs increase gastric motility and how do they exert their effects?
➤ **Metoclopramide:** This D$_2$ receptor antagonist also exerts prokinetic effects by stimulation of muscarinic, 5-HT$_3$ and 5-HT$_4$ receptors in the GIT. It causes relaxation of the pyloric sphincter, increased peristalsis in the jejunum and duodenum and increases stomach emptying. This may contribute to its antiemetic actions. Metoclopramide is often used on ICU for the treatment of gastric stasis and ileus.

➤ **Domperidone:** This D_2 receptor antagonist is primarily an antiemetic but it also increases gastrointestinal motility. It is used in the treatment of postprandial bloating, reflux and belching.
➤ **Neostigmine:** This acetylcholinesterase inhibitor increases the availability of acetylcholine (ACh) at the myenteric plexus, resulting in increased gut motility, salivation, gastric secretions and sphincter tone. It is occasionally used on the ICU to treat refractory constipation.
➤ **Cisapride:** This prokinetic agent acts at $5\text{-}HT_4$ receptors enhancing ACh release at the myenteric plexus. This increases sphincter tone and peristalsis and the drug used to be prescribed for reflux oesophagitis. It has now been withdrawn in the UK because it causes long Q-T syndrome, VT, VF and torsades de pointes.

Which drugs inhibit gastric motility and how do they exert their effects?
➤ **Antimuscarinic agents** (e.g. atropine and hyoscine):
  • An increase in parasympathetic tone in the GIT promotes 'resting and digesting'. Antimuscarinic drugs antagonise the muscarinic M_3 receptors, decreasing GIT motility, saliva production, gastric secretions and lower oesophageal sphincter tone.
➤ **Opioids:**
  • Morphine and other opioids are agonists at the MOP receptors in the myenteric plexus. Stimulation of MOP receptors leads to hyperpolarisation of cells, which reduces stomach emptying, decreases gut motility and increases intestinal transit time. They also decrease gastric, biliary and pancreatic secretions. Opioids cause constipation and commonly cause nausea and vomiting by their stimulation of opioid receptors at the CTZ.

CYCLIZINE

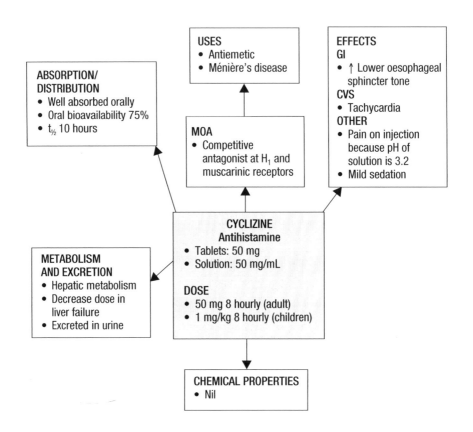

USES
- Antiemetic
- Ménière's disease

EFFECTS
GI
- ↑ Lower oesophageal sphincter tone

CVS
- Tachycardia

OTHER
- Pain on injection because pH of solution is 3.2
- Mild sedation

ABSORPTION/ DISTRIBUTION
- Well absorbed orally
- Oral bioavailability 75%
- $t_{1/2}$ 10 hours

MOA
- Competitive antagonist at H_1 and muscarinic receptors

CYCLIZINE
Antihistamine
- Tablets: 50 mg
- Solution: 50 mg/mL

DOSE
- 50 mg 8 hourly (adult)
- 1 mg/kg 8 hourly (children)

METABOLISM AND EXCRETION
- Hepatic metabolism
- Decrease dose in liver failure
- Excreted in urine

CHEMICAL PROPERTIES
- Nil

CHLORPROMAZINE

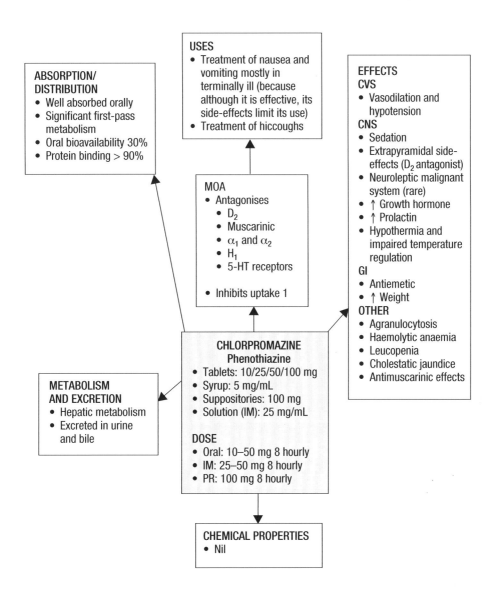

ABSORPTION/DISTRIBUTION
- Well absorbed orally
- Significant first-pass metabolism
- Oral bioavailability 30%
- Protein binding > 90%

USES
- Treatment of nausea and vomiting mostly in terminally ill (because although it is effective, its side-effects limit its use)
- Treatment of hiccoughs

EFFECTS
CVS
- Vasodilation and hypotension

CNS
- Sedation
- Extrapyramidal side-effects (D_2 antagonist)
- Neuroleptic malignant system (rare)
- ↑ Growth hormone
- ↑ Prolactin
- Hypothermia and impaired temperature regulation

GI
- Antiemetic
- ↑ Weight

OTHER
- Agranulocytosis
- Haemolytic anaemia
- Leucopenia
- Cholestatic jaundice
- Antimuscarinic effects

MOA
- Antagonises
  - D_2
  - Muscarinic
  - α_1 and α_2
  - H_1
  - 5-HT receptors
- Inhibits uptake 1

METABOLISM AND EXCRETION
- Hepatic metabolism
- Excreted in urine and bile

CHLORPROMAZINE
Phenothiazine
- Tablets: 10/25/50/100 mg
- Syrup: 5 mg/mL
- Suppositories: 100 mg
- Solution (IM): 25 mg/mL

DOSE
- Oral: 10–50 mg 8 hourly
- IM: 25–50 mg 8 hourly
- PR: 100 mg 8 hourly

CHEMICAL PROPERTIES
- Nil

DOMPERIDONE

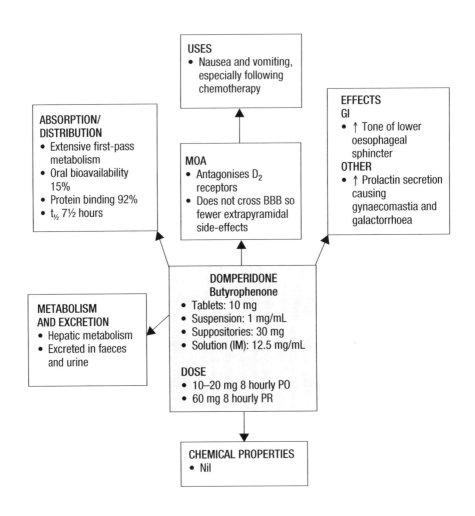

USES
- Nausea and vomiting, especially following chemotherapy

ABSORPTION/ DISTRIBUTION
- Extensive first-pass metabolism
- Oral bioavailability 15%
- Protein binding 92%
- $t_{1/2}$ 7½ hours

MOA
- Antagonises D_2 receptors
- Does not cross BBB so fewer extrapyramidal side-effects

EFFECTS
GI
- ↑ Tone of lower oesophageal sphincter

OTHER
- ↑ Prolactin secretion causing gynaecomastia and galactorrhoea

METABOLISM AND EXCRETION
- Hepatic metabolism
- Excreted in faeces and urine

DOMPERIDONE
Butyrophenone
- Tablets: 10 mg
- Suspension: 1 mg/mL
- Suppositories: 30 mg
- Solution (IM): 12.5 mg/mL

DOSE
- 10–20 mg 8 hourly PO
- 60 mg 8 hourly PR

CHEMICAL PROPERTIES
- Nil

METOCLOPRAMIDE

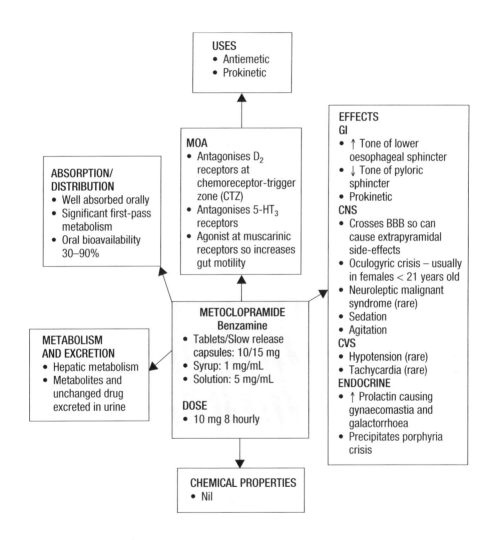

USES
- Antiemetic
- Prokinetic

MOA
- Antagonises D_2 receptors at chemoreceptor-trigger zone (CTZ)
- Antagonises $5\text{-}HT_3$ receptors
- Agonist at muscarinic receptors so increases gut motility

ABSORPTION/ DISTRIBUTION
- Well absorbed orally
- Significant first-pass metabolism
- Oral bioavailability 30–90%

EFFECTS
GI
- ↑ Tone of lower oesophageal sphincter
- ↓ Tone of pyloric sphincter
- Prokinetic

CNS
- Crosses BBB so can cause extrapyramidal side-effects
- Oculogyric crisis – usually in females < 21 years old
- Neuroleptic malignant syndrome (rare)
- Sedation
- Agitation

CVS
- Hypotension (rare)
- Tachycardia (rare)

ENDOCRINE
- ↑ Prolactin causing gynaecomastia and galactorrhoea
- Precipitates porphyria crisis

METOCLOPRAMIDE
Benzamine
- Tablets/Slow release capsules: 10/15 mg
- Syrup: 1 mg/mL
- Solution: 5 mg/mL

DOSE
- 10 mg 8 hourly

METABOLISM AND EXCRETION
- Hepatic metabolism
- Metabolites and unchanged drug excreted in urine

CHEMICAL PROPERTIES
- Nil

ONDANSETRON

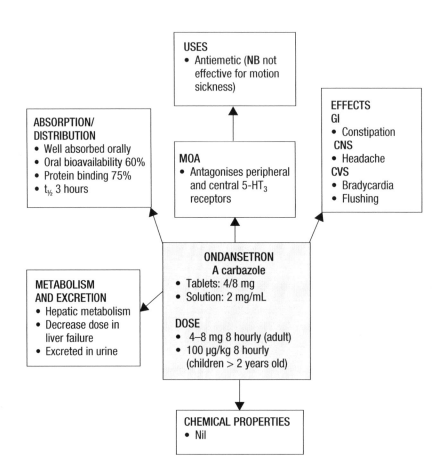

USES
- Antiemetic (NB not effective for motion sickness)

EFFECTS
GI
- Constipation

CNS
- Headache

CVS
- Bradycardia
- Flushing

ABSORPTION/ DISTRIBUTION
- Well absorbed orally
- Oral bioavailability 60%
- Protein binding 75%
- $t_{1/2}$ 3 hours

MOA
- Antagonises peripheral and central 5-HT$_3$ receptors

ONDANSETRON
A carbazole
- Tablets: 4/8 mg
- Solution: 2 mg/mL

DOSE
- 4–8 mg 8 hourly (adult)
- 100 µg/kg 8 hourly (children > 2 years old)

METABOLISM AND EXCRETION
- Hepatic metabolism
- Decrease dose in liver failure
- Excreted in urine

CHEMICAL PROPERTIES
- Nil

PROCHLORPERAZINE

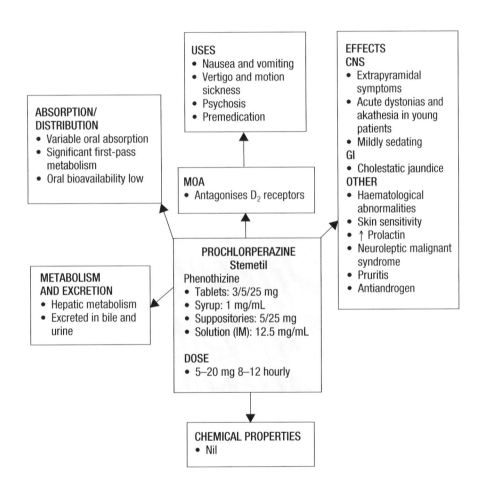

USES
- Nausea and vomiting
- Vertigo and motion sickness
- Psychosis
- Premedication

EFFECTS
CNS
- Extrapyramidal symptoms
- Acute dystonias and akathesia in young patients
- Mildly sedating

GI
- Cholestatic jaundice

OTHER
- Haematological abnormalities
- Skin sensitivity
- ↑ Prolactin
- Neuroleptic malignant syndrome
- Pruritis
- Antiandrogen

ABSORPTION/ DISTRIBUTION
- Variable oral absorption
- Significant first-pass metabolism
- Oral bioavailability low

MOA
- Antagonises D_2 receptors

PROCHLORPERAZINE
Stemetil
Phenothizine
- Tablets: 3/5/25 mg
- Syrup: 1 mg/mL
- Suppositories: 5/25 mg
- Solution (IM): 12.5 mg/mL

DOSE
- 5–20 mg 8–12 hourly

METABOLISM AND EXCRETION
- Hepatic metabolism
- Excreted in bile and urine

CHEMICAL PROPERTIES
- Nil

CHAPTER 24

Antiarrhythmic drugs

Describe the classification of antiarrhythmic drugs

Antiarrhythmics are classified traditionally according to the Vaughn–Williams system (*see* Table 1.34). This system is not particularly useful as many drugs are not included (e.g. adenosine and digoxin) and many could fit into more than one category (e.g. amiodarone and sotalol). However, the examiners still expect you to know it. Many of the drugs have actions other than just their antiarrhythmic ones, and they are discussed in more detail in their relevant spider diagrams.

When answering questions on antiarrhythmics it is best to draw the graph of the nodal and myocyte action potentials to illustrate your answers.

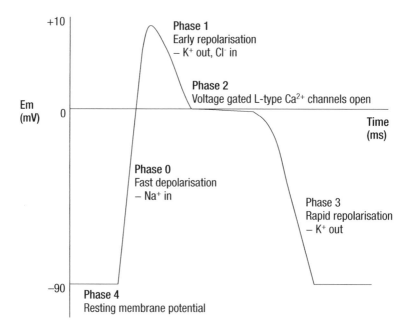

The Vaughn–Williams classification of antiarrhythmics

FIGURE 1.32 Cardiac myocyte action potential (AP)

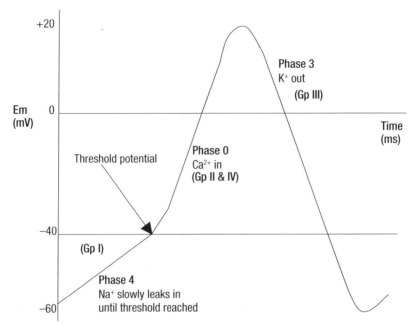

FIGURE 1.33 Sinoatrial node action potential (AP)

TABLE 1.34 Vaughn-Williams classification of antiarrhythmics

Class	Mechanism	Drug
Ia	Blocks fast Na$^+$ channels in cardiac myocytes. ↑ Refractory period	Quinidine, Procainamide, Disopyramide
Ib	Blocks fast Na$^+$ channels in cardiac myocytes. ↓ Refractory period	Lignocaine, Phenytoin, Mexiletine
Ic	Blocks fast Na$^+$ channels in cardiac myocytes. No effect on refractory period	Flecainide, Propafenone
II	β-adrenoreceptor blockade	Atenolol, Propranolol, Esmolol
III	K$^+$ channel blockade	Amiodarone, Sotalol, Bretylium
IV	Ca^{2+} channel blockade	Verapamil, Diltiazem

Groups II–IV refer to the class of antiarrhythmic agents which exert their effect at the various phases of the sinoatrial node action potential.

How do class I drugs exert their effects?
Refer to the cardiac myocyte AP graph (Figure 1.32):
   The sodium channel blockers exert their effects by blocking fast Na$^+$ channels, therefore reducing the influx of Na$^+$ into cardiac myocytes and increasing the time it takes the cell to reach threshold potential. By doing this they decrease the slope of Phase 0 of the AP, and decrease cardiac conduction velocity. For this reason, they are effective at abolishing re-entrant arrhythmias. These fast Na$^+$ channels are not found in nodal tissue, where Phase 0 depolarisation results from the influx of Ca^{2+} ions.
   Class I drugs are further sub-classified according to their effects on the refractory period (RP) of the myocyte. Class I drugs may prolong or decrease the time taken for repolarisation, and therefore the RP, by their action on the K$^+$ channels responsible for Phase 3 of the AP.

How do class II drugs exert their effects?
Refer to the sinoatrial node AP graph (Figure 1.33):

β blockers are antagonists at β adrenoceptors and so decrease sympathetic tone on the heart, which reduces the slope of Phase 4 of the AP.

β adrenoceptors are found in nodal, conducting and myocardial tissues and are coupled, via G proteins, to Ca^{2+} channels that open when the receptor is activated. In the cardiac tissues there are relatively more $β_1$ than $β_2$ adrenoceptors, and the newer generations of β blockers are much more cardioselective, ($β_1 > β_2$). Blocking β adrenoceptors causes a decrease in Ca^{2+} flux into cells and so reduces the slope of Phase 0 of the AP. A decrease in Ca^{2+} influx causes:

➤ decrease in heart rate (chronotropy)
➤ decrease in contractility (ionotropy) as less Ca^{2+} is available to the sarcomeres in the myocytes.

β blockers also inhibit the action of myosin light chain kinase and so they decrease the heart's relaxation rate (lusitropy).

How do class III drugs exert their effects?
Refer to the sinoatrial node AP graph (Figure 1.33):

Class III antiarrhythmics block K^+ channels, decreasing K^+ flux out of the cells which delays repolarisation both in nodal tissue and in the cardiac myocytes. This decreases the slope of phase 3 of the AP, which leads to an increase in the cells' refractory period and hence reduces its arrhythmogenicity.

How do class IV drugs exert their effects?
Refer to the sinoatrial nodal AP graph (Figure 1.33):

Class IV antiarrhythmics block L-type Ca^{2+} channels, while leaving T, N and P type channels unaffected. L-type channels are widespread throughout the cardiovascular system. T-type are structurally similar to L and are present in the cardiac cells that have T-tubule systems, e.g. SA node and some vascular tissues. N-type are found in nerve cells and P in the Purkinje fibres. L-type Ca^{2+} channels are responsible for the plateau phase of the cardiac action potential. Class IV drugs decrease the slope of Phase 0 of the nodal AP, decreasing heart rate. These channels are also found in cardiac myocytes and blood vessels and decreasing Ca^{2+} flux reduces cardiac conduction velocity and contractility.

What are the main differences between verapamil and nifedipine?
Verapamil is a racemic mixture whose L isomer has a high affinity for the L-type Ca^{2+} channels at the SA and AV nodes. This results in slowing of conduction through the pacemaker cells, a decrease in heart rate and an increase in the RP. Verapamil's effect on cardiac contractility and vascular tone is less marked though it does cause some coronary artery vasodilation.

Nifedipine has little effect on the SA or AV nodes but causes a marked decrease in arterial tone. For this reason it is used for arterial spasm in coronary angiography, Raynaud's phenomenon, hypertension and angina.

Which agents would you use to treat an SVT and a VT?

SVTs can be treated with drugs from groups:	VTs can be treated with drugs from groups:
Ia	Ia
Ic	Ib
III (but not bretylium)	Ic
IV	III

QUINIDINE

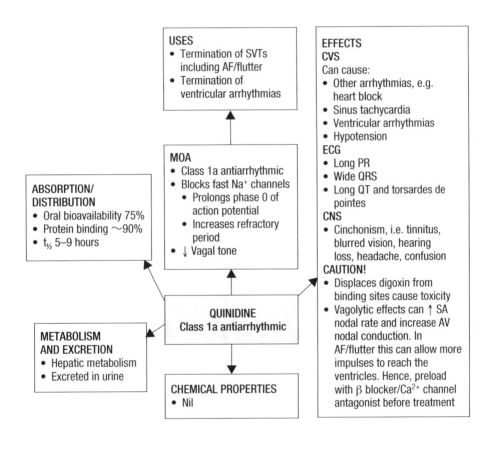

USES
- Termination of SVTs including AF/flutter
- Termination of ventricular arrhythmias

MOA
- Class 1a antiarrhythmic
- Blocks fast Na^+ channels
  - Prolongs phase 0 of action potential
  - Increases refractory period
- ↓ Vagal tone

ABSORPTION/ DISTRIBUTION
- Oral bioavailability 75%
- Protein binding ~90%
- $t_{1/2}$ 5–9 hours

QUINIDINE
Class 1a antiarrhythmic

METABOLISM AND EXCRETION
- Hepatic metabolism
- Excreted in urine

CHEMICAL PROPERTIES
- Nil

EFFECTS
CVS
Can cause:
- Other arrhythmias, e.g. heart block
- Sinus tachycardia
- Ventricular arrhythmias
- Hypotension

ECG
- Long PR
- Wide QRS
- Long QT and torsardes de pointes

CNS
- Cinchonism, i.e. tinnitus, blurred vision, hearing loss, headache, confusion

CAUTION!
- Displaces digoxin from binding sites cause toxicity
- Vagolytic effects can ↑ SA nodal rate and increase AV nodal conduction. In AF/flutter this can allow more impulses to reach the ventricles. Hence, preload with β blocker/Ca^{2+} channel antagonist before treatment

LIGNOCAINE

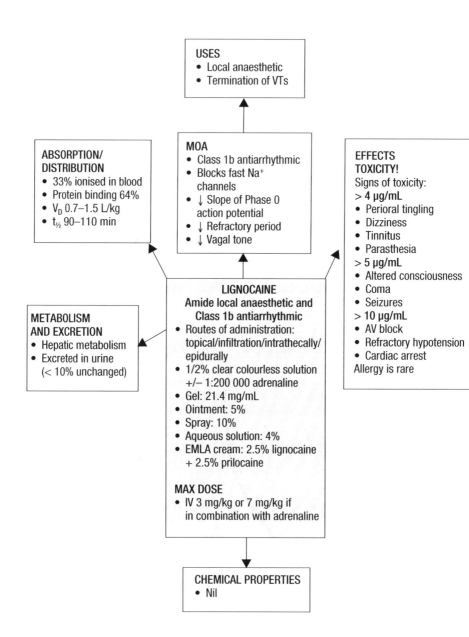

USES
- Local anaesthetic
- Termination of VTs

ABSORPTION/
DISTRIBUTION
- 33% ionised in blood
- Protein binding 64%
- V_D 0.7–1.5 L/kg
- $t_{1/2}$ 90–110 min

MOA
- Class 1b antiarrhythmic
- Blocks fast Na^+
  channels
- ↓ Slope of Phase 0
  action potential
- ↓ Refractory period
- ↓ Vagal tone

EFFECTS
TOXICITY!
Signs of toxicity:
> 4 µg/mL
- Perioral tingling
- Dizziness
- Tinnitus
- Parasthesia
> 5 µg/mL
- Altered consciousness
- Coma
- Seizures
> 10 µg/mL
- AV block
- Refractory hypotension
- Cardiac arrest
Allergy is rare

METABOLISM
AND EXCRETION
- Hepatic metabolism
- Excreted in urine
  (< 10% unchanged)

LIGNOCAINE
Amide local anaesthetic and
Class 1b antiarrhythmic
- Routes of administration:
  topical/infiltration/intrathecally/
  epidurally
- 1/2% clear colourless solution
  +/− 1:200 000 adrenaline
- Gel: 21.4 mg/mL
- Ointment: 5%
- Spray: 10%
- Aqueous solution: 4%
- EMLA cream: 2.5% lignocaine
  + 2.5% prilocaine

MAX DOSE
- IV 3 mg/kg or 7 mg/kg if
  in combination with adrenaline

CHEMICAL PROPERTIES
- Nil

FLECAINIDE

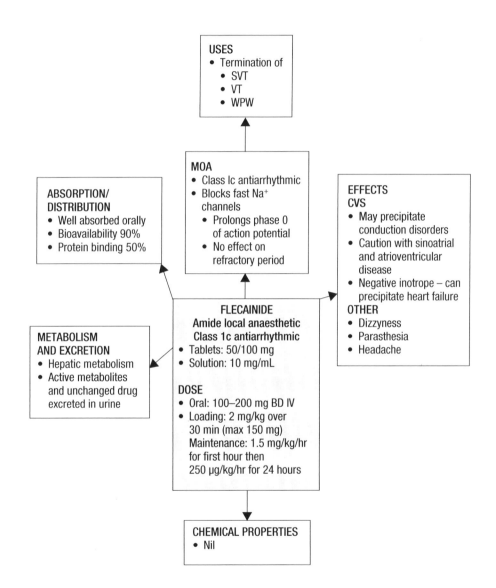

USES
- Termination of
  - SVT
  - VT
  - WPW

MOA
- Class Ic antiarrhythmic
- Blocks fast Na^+ channels
  - Prolongs phase 0 of action potential
  - No effect on refractory period

ABSORPTION/ DISTRIBUTION
- Well absorbed orally
- Bioavailability 90%
- Protein binding 50%

EFFECTS
CVS
- May precipitate conduction disorders
- Caution with sinoatrial and atrioventricular disease
- Negative inotrope – can precipitate heart failure

OTHER
- Dizzyness
- Parasthesia
- Headache

FLECAINIDE
Amide local anaesthetic
Class 1c antiarrhythmic
- Tablets: 50/100 mg
- Solution: 10 mg/mL

DOSE
- Oral: 100–200 mg BD IV
- Loading: 2 mg/kg over 30 min (max 150 mg) Maintenance: 1.5 mg/kg/hr for first hour then 250 µg/kg/hr for 24 hours

METABOLISM AND EXCRETION
- Hepatic metabolism
- Active metabolites and unchanged drug excreted in urine

CHEMICAL PROPERTIES
- Nil

AMIODARONE

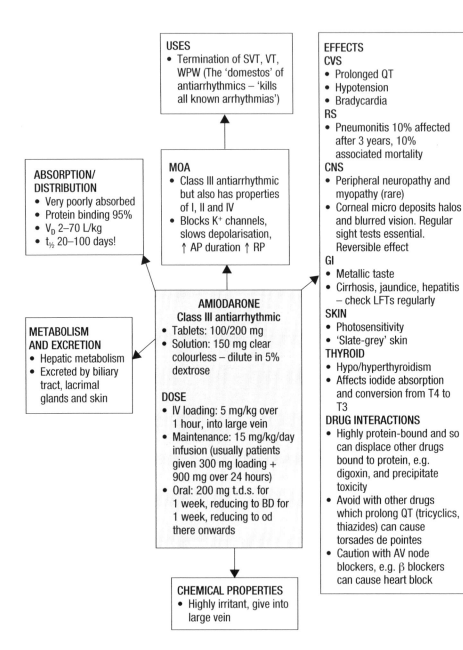

USES
- Termination of SVT, VT, WPW (The 'domestos' of antiarrhythmics – 'kills all known arrhythmias')

ABSORPTION/ DISTRIBUTION
- Very poorly absorbed
- Protein binding 95%
- V_D 2–70 L/kg
- $t_{1/2}$ 20–100 days!

MOA
- Class III antiarrhythmic but also has properties of I, II and IV
- Blocks K^+ channels, slows depolarisation, ↑ AP duration ↑ RP

METABOLISM AND EXCRETION
- Hepatic metabolism
- Excreted by biliary tract, lacrimal glands and skin

**AMIODARONE
Class III antiarrhythmic**
- Tablets: 100/200 mg
- Solution: 150 mg clear colourless – dilute in 5% dextrose

DOSE
- IV loading: 5 mg/kg over 1 hour, into large vein
- Maintenance: 15 mg/kg/day infusion (usually patients given 300 mg loading + 900 mg over 24 hours)
- Oral: 200 mg t.d.s. for 1 week, reducing to BD for 1 week, reducing to od there onwards

CHEMICAL PROPERTIES
- Highly irritant, give into large vein

EFFECTS
CVS
- Prolonged QT
- Hypotension
- Bradycardia

RS
- Pneumonitis 10% affected after 3 years, 10% associated mortality

CNS
- Peripheral neuropathy and myopathy (rare)
- Corneal micro deposits halos and blurred vision. Regular sight tests essential. Reversible effect

GI
- Metallic taste
- Cirrhosis, jaundice, hepatitis – check LFTs regularly

SKIN
- Photosensitivity
- 'Slate-grey' skin

THYROID
- Hypo/hyperthyroidism
- Affects iodide absorption and conversion from T4 to T3

DRUG INTERACTIONS
- Highly protein-bound and so can displace other drugs bound to protein, e.g. digoxin, and precipitate toxicity
- Avoid with other drugs which prolong QT (tricyclics, thiazides) can cause torsades de pointes
- Caution with AV node blockers, e.g. β blockers can cause heart block

DIGOXIN

USES
- To slow rate of AF and flutter
- Ionotrope in cardiac failure

MOA
- Binds to and inhibits Na$^+$/K$^+$ATPase pump. This causes rise in intracellular [Na$^+$]. This decreases extrusion of Ca^{2+} by Na$^+$/Ca^{2+} exchange pump, because this relies on high concentration gradient of Na$^+$ across cell membrane (which is reduced).
- ↑ intracellular Ca^{2+} causes ↑ **contractility**
- ↓ intracellular K$^+$ causes ↓ conduction in SA & AV node, **slowing HR**
- Increases vagal tone, so ↑ AV conduction time

EFFECTS
CVS
Arrhythmias and conduction abnormalities:
- Premature ventricular contraction
- Bigeminy
- AV block – all types
- Junctional rhythm
- Atrial/ventricular tachycardia
ECG
- Long PR (toxicity)
- 'Inverted tick' (toxicity)
- Flat T wave (at therapeutic level)
- Short QT (at therapeutic level)
OTHER
- Anorexia
- Nausea and vomiting
- Diarrhoea
- Headache
- Lethargy
- Visual disturbances of red-green perception
- Rashes
- Eosinophilia
- Gynaecomastia
Plasma levels:
- ↑ By amiodarone, erythromycin, captopril
- ↓ By antacids, phenytoin, metoclopramide

ABSORPTION/ DISTRIBUTION
- Oral bioavailability > 70%
- Protein binding 25%
- V$_D$ 5–10 L/kg
- t$_½$ 35 hours, ↑↑↑ in renal failure

METABOLISM AND EXCRETION
- Minimal hepatic metabolism
- Excreted unchanged in urine

DIGOXIN
Glycoside extracted from foxglove leaves (*digitalis lanata*)
- Tablets: 62.5–250 µg
- Colourless solution: 100–250 µg/mL

DOSE
- Loading: 500 µg followed by 500 µg or 250 µg 6 hours later (depending on patient's size)
- Maintenance: 62.5–500 µg/day
- Therapeutic range: 1–2 µg/L

TOXICITY
- **TOXIC** at [plasma] > 2.5 µg/L serious effects not usually seen at < 10 µg/L
- > 30 µg/L fatal
- Treat bradycardia with atropine or pacing
- Treat ventricular arrhythmias with phenytoin
- 'Digibind' antidote available (IgG antibody fragments against digoxin, bind and the complex is removed by kidneys), but very expensive. Use if > 20 µg/L, life threatening arrhythmias, uncontrolled hyperkalaemia
- Digibind can cause anaphylaxis

VERAPAMIL

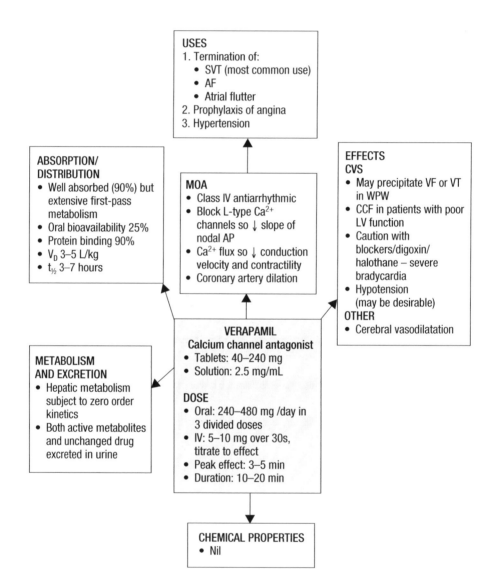

USES
1. Termination of:
   - SVT (most common use)
   - AF
   - Atrial flutter
2. Prophylaxis of angina
3. Hypertension

ABSORPTION/ DISTRIBUTION
- Well absorbed (90%) but extensive first-pass metabolism
- Oral bioavailability 25%
- Protein binding 90%
- V_D 3–5 L/kg
- $t_{1/2}$ 3–7 hours

MOA
- Class IV antiarrhythmic
- Block L-type Ca^{2+} channels so ↓ slope of nodal AP
- Ca^{2+} flux so ↓ conduction velocity and contractility
- Coronary artery dilation

EFFECTS
CVS
- May precipitate VF or VT in WPW
- CCF in patients with poor LV function
- Caution with blockers/digoxin/ halothane – severe bradycardia
- Hypotension (may be desirable)

OTHER
- Cerebral vasodilatation

VERAPAMIL
Calcium channel antagonist
- Tablets: 40–240 mg
- Solution: 2.5 mg/mL

DOSE
- Oral: 240–480 mg /day in 3 divided doses
- IV: 5–10 mg over 30s, titrate to effect
- Peak effect: 3–5 min
- Duration: 10–20 min

METABOLISM AND EXCRETION
- Hepatic metabolism subject to zero order kinetics
- Both active metabolites and unchanged drug excreted in urine

CHEMICAL PROPERTIES
- Nil

β BLOCKERS

EFFECTS
CVS
- Negative inotrope and chronotrope so:
  - ↑ Time in diastole and coronary artery perfusion
  - ↓ Cardiac oxygen requirements BUT, may worsen performance of failing ventricle
- ↓ BP
  - ↓ HR and CO
  - ↓ Renin secretion by β_1 inhibition at juxtaglomerular apparatus BUT: beware in peripheral vascular disease as inhibition of β_2 receptors causes some constriction which may further compromise circulation in peripheries.

RS
- Bronchospasm, worse in susceptible patients so give cardioselective drugs in asthma/COPD and give test dose of short acting drug, e.g. esmolol/metoprolol

CNS
- Cross BBB can cause:
  - Hallucinations
  - Nightmares
  - Depression
  - Fatigue
  - ↓ Intraocular pressure

GI
- Dry mouth
- GI upset

METABOLIC
Non-selective agents can:
- ↑ Resting BM in diabetics
- mask symptoms of hypoglycaemia (sweating, tachycardia, etc.)
- ↑ Triglycerides and ↓ HDL

USES
- Hypertension
- Angina and MI
- Tachycardias
- Obtund reflex hypertension during laryngoscopy, e.g. esmolol
- In phaeochromocytoma – pre-op stabilisation
- HOCM
- Anxiety
- Glaucoma
- Migraine prophylaxis

ABSORPTION/ DISTRIBUTION
- Varying lipid solubility of different agents
- Low lipid solubility, e.g. atenolol = poorly absorbed from gut
- Higher lipid solubility, e.g. metoprolol = well absorbed, but cross BBB and ↑ CNS side-effects
- Variable protein binding

MOA
- All competitive antagonists at β adrenoreceptor
- Some have intrinsic sympathomimetic activity
- Varying receptor affinity (see box below)

METABOLISM AND EXCRETION
- Low lipid solubility = minimal hepatic metabolism and excreted unchanged in urine
- High lipid solubility = hepatic metabolism

β BLOCKERS
(Class II antiarrhythmic)

RECEPTOR SELECTIVITY
Aim to block β1 but not β2 receptors.
'Cardioselective' drugs:
- Atenolol
- Esmolol (ultra-short acting)
- Metoprolol (short acting)
- Bisoprolol
- Carvedilol

NB all will act on β2 if dose high enough

ADENOSINE

USES
- To differentiate between SVT (rate slows) and VT (rate doesn't slow)
- If tachyarrhythmia is re-entrant, it may terminate it
- To differentiate between atrial fibrillation and flutter, by slowing ECG trace for analysis

MOA
- Binds to **adenosine (A1) receptors** coupled with K^+ channels that open, to hyperpolarised membrane
- A1 receptors only found in sinoatrial and atrioventricular nodes so adenosine selectively decreases conduction velocity in the nodes (negative dromotropic effect)
- Also decreases cAMP mediated catecholamine stimulation of ventricles (negative chronotropic effect)

ABSORPTION/ DISTRIBUTION
- $t_{1/2} < 10$ s

METABOLISM AND EXCRETION
- Deamination in plasma and red blood cells

ADENOSINE
Naturally occurring purine nucleoside
- Colourless solution: 3 mg/mL

DOSE
- Give incremental doses at 1 min intervals until desired effect achieved 6 mg/12 mg/ 18 mg
- Give as fast bolus into large vein

EFFECTS
CVS
- No clinically significant effects on BP when given as described

OTHER
- ↑Pulmonary vascular resistance
- SOB, flushing and chest discomfort
- Bronchospasm in asthmatics
- Sense of impending doom. (Patients genuinely feel like they're going to die. Warn them of this and support them through the feeling. It only lasts a few seconds.)

CHEMICAL PROPERTIES
- Nil

CHAPTER 25

Antihypertensive agents

What are the major categories of antihypertensive drugs and what are their mechanism of actions?

$$MAP = CO \times SVR$$
$$CO = SV \times HR \text{ (SV depends on preload, contractility and afterload)}$$

Antihypertensive agents will produce their effect by either modulating cardiac output (CO), systemic vascular resistance (SVR) or both. The easiest way to categorise antihypertensive agents is according to their site of action:

Heart:
➤ **β-blockers** – Competitive antagonists at β-adrenoceptors with varying degrees of receptor selectivity. Negative inotropic and chronotropic effects reduce CO while antagonism of the renal β_1 adrenoceptors reduces sympathetically mediated release of renin.
  - **Atenolol, esmolol and metoprolol** – Cardioselective (i.e. act only on β_1 adrenoceptors at normal doses).
  - **Propranolol** – Non-cardioselective (i.e. acts at both β_1 and β_2 adrenoceptors).
  - **Labetalol** – Non-cardioselective and has antagonistic action at α_1-adrenoceptors (ratio of α_1: β blockade depends on the route of administration: oral = 1:3 and IV =1:7).

Blood vessels:
➤ **Directly acting vasodilators** – Produce NO, which acts on G-protein coupled receptors activating guanylate cyclase and increasing intracellular cGMP levels to cause vasodilatation.
  - **Sodium nitroprusside and hydralazine** – Produce vasodilatation of both arterial and venous vessels. Arterial vasodilatation reduces SVR while venous vasodilatation increases venous capacitance and reduces preload.
  - **Glyceryl trinitrate and isosorbide mononitrate** – Produce vasodilatation of primarily the venous vessels. This increases venous capacitance and reduces preload.
➤ **Indirectly acting vasodilators** – Reduce SVR and preload by various mechanisms.
  - **Calcium channel blockers** (e.g. amlodipine) – Antagonists at L-type calcium channel located in vascular smooth muscle.
  - **α-blockers** (e.g. prazosin) – Antagonists at α_1-adrenoceptors causing vasodilatation of both arterial and venous vessels.
  - **Potassium channel activators** (e.g. nicorandil) – Activators of ATP-sensitive K^+ channels within arterioles causing hyperpolarisation, reduced intracellular Ca^{2+} levels and hence arteriolar vasodilatation. Venous vessels are also relaxed by activation of guanylate cyclase by the nitrate moiety within nicorandil.
  - **Magnesium** – This is a natural antagonist to calcium.

Kidney:
➤ **Diuretics** – Reduce plasma volume (which reduces preload and CO) and some produce arteriolar vasodilatation reducing SVR (e.g. thiazide and loop diuretics). *See* Chapter 26, 'Diuretics'.
➤ **Agents effecting the renin-angiotensin-aldosterone system** – see later
  • Angiotensin converting enzyme inhibitors, ACEI (e.g. ramipril).
  • Angiotensin II receptor antagonists (e.g. losartan).

Central nervous system:
➤ **Centrally acting drugs** (e.g. clonidine and methyldopa) – Stimulate central inhibitory presynaptic α_2-adrenoceptors causing reduced noradrenaline release and hence reduced centrally mediated sympathetic outflow.
➤ **Ganglion blockers** (e.g. trimetaphan) – Competitive antagonists at nACh receptors located in parasympathetic and sympathetic ganglia.

Briefly explain the renin-angiotensin-aldosterone system (RAAS)
RAAS system is intricately involved in the regulation of blood pressure. Renin is released from the juxtaglomerular apparatus in response to low renal perfusion, reduced Na^+ at the macula densa or sympathetic stimulation via renal β_1 adrenoceptors. Renin converts angiotensinogen, which is produced by the liver, into angiotensin I. Angiotensin I is then converted into angiotensin II in the lung via the action of angiotensin converting enzyme (ACE). Angiotensin II produces a multitude of effects including peripheral vasoconstriction, aldosterone release from the adrenal cortex, increased thirst sensation and increased ADH (also known as vasopressin) and ACTH release from the hypothalamo-pituitary axis.

What are some of the commoner side-effects of antihypertensive agents?
➤ **β-blockers** – Unwanted side-effects come from antagonism of β_2 adrenoceptors, which may cause bronchospasm and peripheral vasoconstriction. Hence these agents are best avoided in patients with COPD and peripheral vascular disease.
➤ **Vasodilators** – Vasodilatation of the capacitance vessels can cause postural hypotension while vasodilatation of cerebral vessels can lead to headaches.
➤ **Diuretics** – Loop and thiazide diuretics can both lead to hyponatraemia, hypokalaemia, hypomagnesaemia and hypochloraemic alkalosis due to their action on renal electrolyte reabsorption. Loop diuretics can also cause ototoxity leading to deafness while thiazide diuretics can cause hyperuricaemia and precipitate gout. Due to the risk of hypokalaemia these agents should be used cautiously with digoxin.
➤ **ACEI** – Under normal conditions angiotensin II maintains renal perfusion by altering the calibre of the efferent arteriole at the glomerulus. However, in the presence of an ACEI this mechanism is lost and renal perfusion pressure may fall leading to renal failures in those individuals who already have impaired renal circulation. Hence these agents are contraindicated in renal artery stenosis. Some patients may experience a persistent cough due to increased bradykinin, which is normally degraded by ACE.

NIMODIPINE

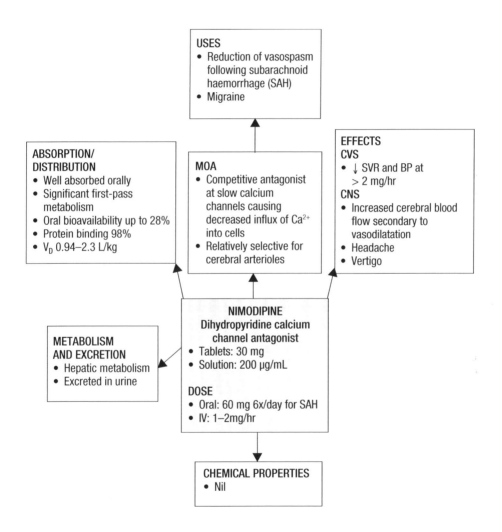

USES
- Reduction of vasospasm following subarachnoid haemorrhage (SAH)
- Migraine

ABSORPTION/ DISTRIBUTION
- Well absorbed orally
- Significant first-pass metabolism
- Oral bioavailability up to 28%
- Protein binding 98%
- V_D 0.94–2.3 L/kg

MOA
- Competitive antagonist at slow calcium channels causing decreased influx of Ca^{2+} into cells
- Relatively selective for cerebral arterioles

EFFECTS
CVS
- ↓ SVR and BP at > 2 mg/hr

CNS
- Increased cerebral blood flow secondary to vasodilatation
- Headache
- Vertigo

METABOLISM AND EXCRETION
- Hepatic metabolism
- Excreted in urine

NIMODIPINE
Dihydropyridine calcium channel antagonist
- Tablets: 30 mg
- Solution: 200 µg/mL

DOSE
- Oral: 60 mg 6x/day for SAH
- IV: 1–2mg/hr

CHEMICAL PROPERTIES
- Nil

NIFEDIPINE

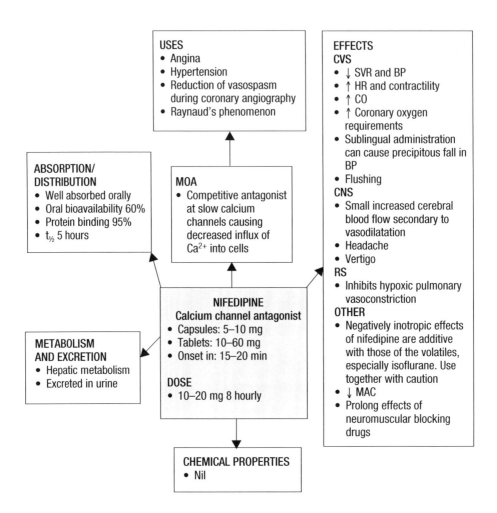

USES
- Angina
- Hypertension
- Reduction of vasospasm during coronary angiography
- Raynaud's phenomenon

ABSORPTION/ DISTRIBUTION
- Well absorbed orally
- Oral bioavailability 60%
- Protein binding 95%
- $t_{1/2}$ 5 hours

MOA
- Competitive antagonist at slow calcium channels causing decreased influx of Ca^{2+} into cells

METABOLISM AND EXCRETION
- Hepatic metabolism
- Excreted in urine

NIFEDIPINE
Calcium channel antagonist
- Capsules: 5–10 mg
- Tablets: 10–60 mg
- Onset in: 15–20 min

DOSE
- 10–20 mg 8 hourly

CHEMICAL PROPERTIES
- Nil

EFFECTS
CVS
- ↓ SVR and BP
- ↑ HR and contractility
- ↑ CO
- ↑ Coronary oxygen requirements
- Sublingual administration can cause precipitous fall in BP
- Flushing

CNS
- Small increased cerebral blood flow secondary to vasodilatation
- Headache
- Vertigo

RS
- Inhibits hypoxic pulmonary vasoconstriction

OTHER
- Negatively inotropic effects of nifedipine are additive with those of the volatiles, especially isoflurane. Use together with caution
- ↓ MAC
- Prolong effects of neuromuscular blocking drugs

CAPTOPRIL

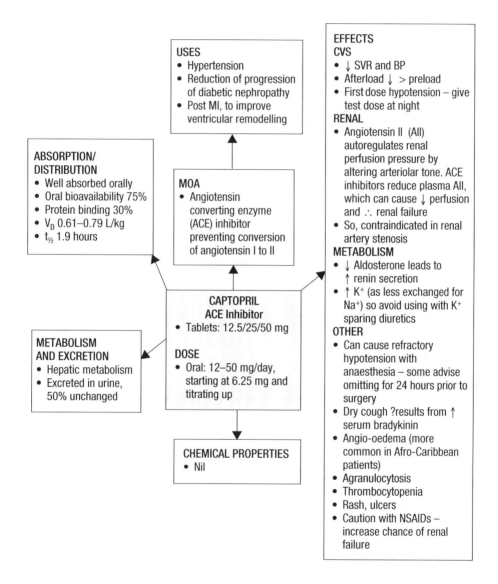

USES
- Hypertension
- Reduction of progression of diabetic nephropathy
- Post MI, to improve ventricular remodelling

ABSORPTION/ DISTRIBUTION
- Well absorbed orally
- Oral bioavailability 75%
- Protein binding 30%
- V_D 0.61–0.79 L/kg
- $t_{1/2}$ 1.9 hours

MOA
- Angiotensin converting enzyme (ACE) inhibitor preventing conversion of angiotensin I to II

CAPTOPRIL
ACE Inhibitor
- Tablets: 12.5/25/50 mg

DOSE
- Oral: 12–50 mg/day, starting at 6.25 mg and titrating up

METABOLISM AND EXCRETION
- Hepatic metabolism
- Excreted in urine, 50% unchanged

CHEMICAL PROPERTIES
- Nil

EFFECTS
CVS
- ↓ SVR and BP
- Afterload ↓ > preload
- First dose hypotension – give test dose at night

RENAL
- Angiotensin II (AII) autoregulates renal perfusion pressure by altering arteriolar tone. ACE inhibitors reduce plasma AII, which can cause ↓ perfusion and ∴ renal failure
- So, contraindicated in renal artery stenosis

METABOLISM
- ↓ Aldosterone leads to ↑ renin secretion
- ↑ K^+ (as less exchanged for Na^+) so avoid using with K^+ sparing diuretics

OTHER
- Can cause refractory hypotension with anaesthesia – some advise omitting for 24 hours prior to surgery
- Dry cough ?results from ↑ serum bradykinin
- Angio-oedema (more common in Afro-Caribbean patients)
- Agranulocytosis
- Thrombocytopenia
- Rash, ulcers
- Caution with NSAIDs – increase chance of renal failure

LOSARTAN

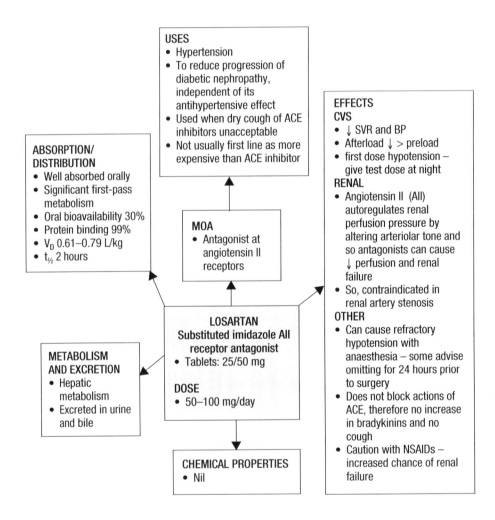

USES
- Hypertension
- To reduce progression of diabetic nephropathy, independent of its antihypertensive effect
- Used when dry cough of ACE inhibitors unacceptable
- Not usually first line as more expensive than ACE inhibitor

ABSORPTION/ DISTRIBUTION
- Well absorbed orally
- Significant first-pass metabolism
- Oral bioavailability 30%
- Protein binding 99%
- V_D 0.61–0.79 L/kg
- $t_{1/2}$ 2 hours

MOA
- Antagonist at angiotensin II receptors

EFFECTS
CVS
- ↓ SVR and BP
- Afterload ↓ > preload
- first dose hypotension – give test dose at night

RENAL
- Angiotensin II (AII) autoregulates renal perfusion pressure by altering arteriolar tone and so antagonists can cause ↓ perfusion and renal failure
- So, contraindicated in renal artery stenosis

OTHER
- Can cause refractory hypotension with anaesthesia – some advise omitting for 24 hours prior to surgery
- Does not block actions of ACE, therefore no increase in bradykinins and no cough
- Caution with NSAIDs – increased chance of renal failure

LOSARTAN
Substituted imidazole AII receptor antagonist
- Tablets: 25/50 mg

DOSE
- 50–100 mg/day

METABOLISM AND EXCRETION
- Hepatic metabolism
- Excreted in urine and bile

CHEMICAL PROPERTIES
- Nil

NICORANDIL

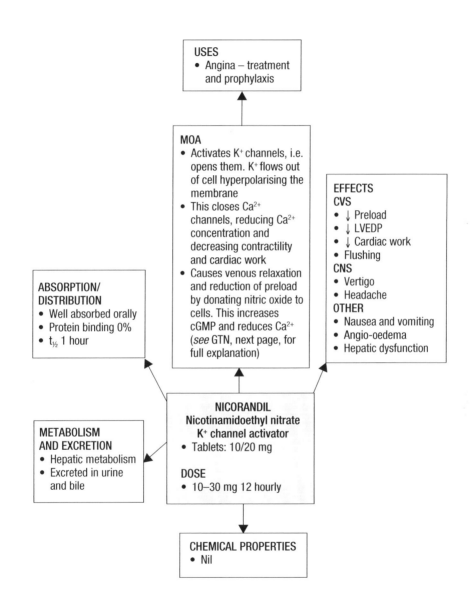

USES
- Angina – treatment and prophylaxis

MOA
- Activates K^+ channels, i.e. opens them. K^+ flows out of cell hyperpolarising the membrane
- This closes Ca^{2+} channels, reducing Ca^{2+} concentration and decreasing contractility and cardiac work
- Causes venous relaxation and reduction of preload by donating nitric oxide to cells. This increases cGMP and reduces Ca^{2+} (*see* GTN, next page, for full explanation)

EFFECTS
CVS
- ↓ Preload
- ↓ LVEDP
- ↓ Cardiac work
- Flushing
CNS
- Vertigo
- Headache
OTHER
- Nausea and vomiting
- Angio-oedema
- Hepatic dysfunction

ABSORPTION/ DISTRIBUTION
- Well absorbed orally
- Protein binding 0%
- $t_{1/2}$ 1 hour

METABOLISM AND EXCRETION
- Hepatic metabolism
- Excreted in urine and bile

NICORANDIL
Nicotinamidoethyl nitrate
K^+ channel activator
- Tablets: 10/20 mg

DOSE
- 10–30 mg 12 hourly

CHEMICAL PROPERTIES
- Nil

GLYCERYL TRINITRITE

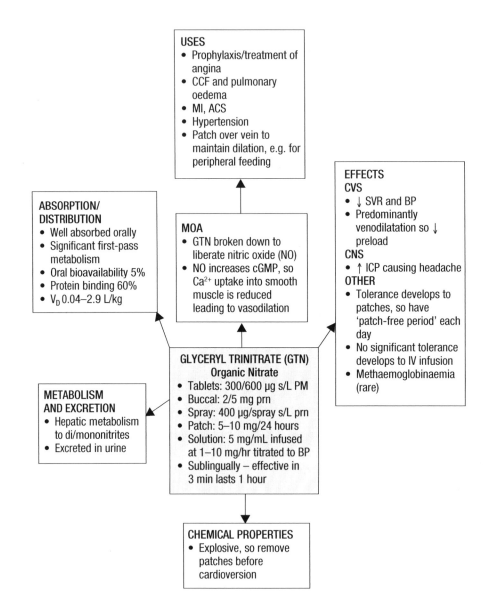

USES
- Prophylaxis/treatment of angina
- CCF and pulmonary oedema
- MI, ACS
- Hypertension
- Patch over vein to maintain dilation, e.g. for peripheral feeding

ABSORPTION/ DISTRIBUTION
- Well absorbed orally
- Significant first-pass metabolism
- Oral bioavailability 5%
- Protein binding 60%
- V_D 0.04–2.9 L/kg

MOA
- GTN broken down to liberate nitric oxide (NO)
- NO increases cGMP, so Ca^{2+} uptake into smooth muscle is reduced leading to vasodilation

EFFECTS
CVS
- ↓ SVR and BP
- Predominantly venodilatation so ↓ preload

CNS
- ↑ ICP causing headache

OTHER
- Tolerance develops to patches, so have 'patch-free period' each day
- No significant tolerance develops to IV infusion
- Methaemoglobinaemia (rare)

GLYCERYL TRINITRATE (GTN)
Organic Nitrate
- Tablets: 300/600 μg s/L PM
- Buccal: 2/5 mg prn
- Spray: 400 μg/spray s/L prn
- Patch: 5–10 mg/24 hours
- Solution: 5 mg/mL infused at 1–10 mg/hr titrated to BP
- Sublingually – effective in 3 min lasts 1 hour

METABOLISM AND EXCRETION
- Hepatic metabolism to di/mononitrites
- Excreted in urine

CHEMICAL PROPERTIES
- Explosive, so remove patches before cardioversion

CLONIDINE

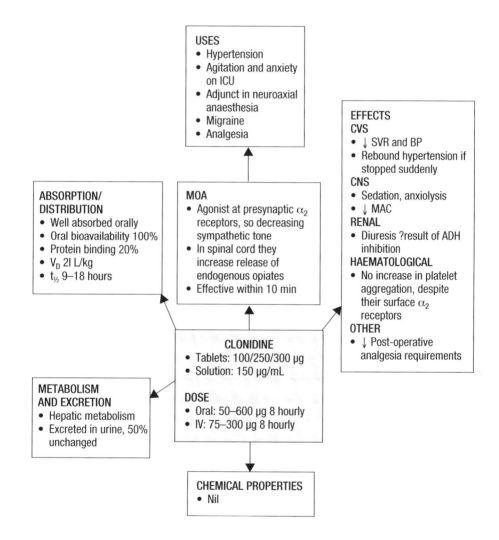

USES
- Hypertension
- Agitation and anxiety on ICU
- Adjunct in neuroaxial anaesthesia
- Migraine
- Analgesia

EFFECTS
CVS
- ↓ SVR and BP
- Rebound hypertension if stopped suddenly
CNS
- Sedation, anxiolysis
- ↓ MAC
RENAL
- Diuresis ?result of ADH inhibition
HAEMATOLOGICAL
- No increase in platelet aggregation, despite their surface α_2 receptors
OTHER
- ↓ Post-operative analgesia requirements

ABSORPTION/ DISTRIBUTION
- Well absorbed orally
- Oral bioavailability 100%
- Protein binding 20%
- V_D 2l L/kg
- $t_{1/2}$ 9–18 hours

MOA
- Agonist at presynaptic α_2 receptors, so decreasing sympathetic tone
- In spinal cord they increase release of endogenous opiates
- Effective within 10 min

CLONIDINE
- Tablets: 100/250/300 µg
- Solution: 150 µg/mL

DOSE
- Oral: 50–600 µg 8 hourly
- IV: 75–300 µg 8 hourly

METABOLISM AND EXCRETION
- Hepatic metabolism
- Excreted in urine, 50% unchanged

CHEMICAL PROPERTIES
- Nil

SODIUM NITROPRUSSIDE

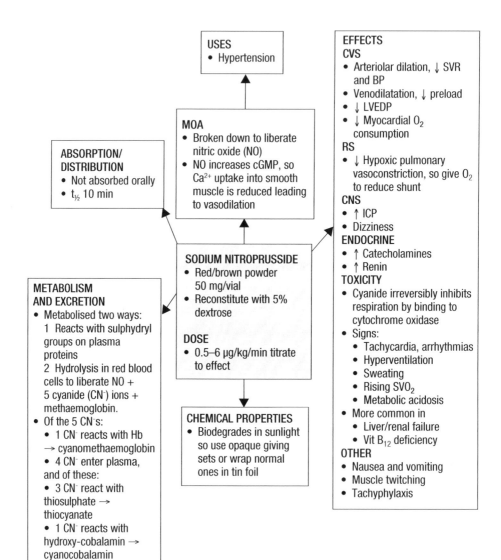

USES
- Hypertension

MOA
- Broken down to liberate nitric oxide (NO)
- NO increases cGMP, so Ca^{2+} uptake into smooth muscle is reduced leading to vasodilation

ABSORPTION/ DISTRIBUTION
- Not absorbed orally
- $t_{1/2}$ 10 min

SODIUM NITROPRUSSIDE
- Red/brown powder 50 mg/vial
- Reconstitute with 5% dextrose

DOSE
- 0.5–6 µg/kg/min titrate to effect

METABOLISM AND EXCRETION
- Metabolised two ways:
  1 Reacts with sulphydryl groups on plasma proteins
  2 Hydrolysis in red blood cells to liberate NO + 5 cyanide (CN^-) ions + methaemoglobin.
- Of the 5 CN^-s:
  - 1 CN^- reacts with Hb → cyanomethaemoglobin
  - 4 CN^- enter plasma, and of these:
  - 3 CN^- react with thiosulphate → thiocyanate
  - 1 CN^- reacts with hydroxy-cobalamin → cyanocobalamin

CHEMICAL PROPERTIES
- Biodegrades in sunlight so use opaque giving sets or wrap normal ones in tin foil

EFFECTS
CVS
- Arteriolar dilation, ↓ SVR and BP
- Venodilatation, ↓ preload
- ↓ LVEDP
- ↓ Myocardial O_2 consumption
RS
- ↓ Hypoxic pulmonary vasoconstriction, so give O_2 to reduce shunt
CNS
- ↑ ICP
- Dizziness
ENDOCRINE
- ↑ Catecholamines
- ↑ Renin
TOXICITY
- Cyanide irreversibly inhibits respiration by binding to cytochrome oxidase
- Signs:
  - Tachycardia, arrhythmias
  - Hyperventilation
  - Sweating
  - Rising SVO_2
  - Metabolic acidosis
- More common in
  - Liver/renal failure
  - Vit B_{12} deficiency
OTHER
- Nausea and vomiting
- Muscle twitching
- Tachyphylaxis

METHYLDOPA

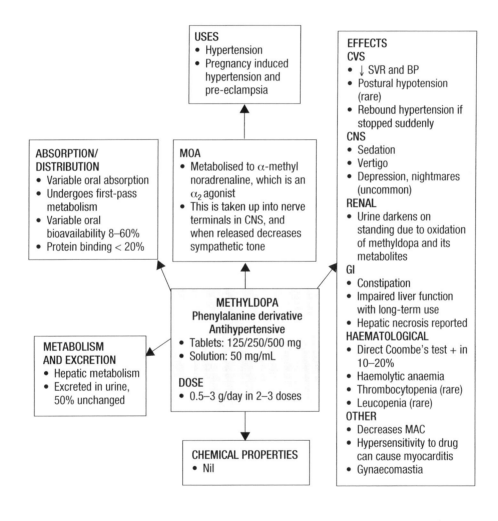

USES
- Hypertension
- Pregnancy induced hypertension and pre-eclampsia

ABSORPTION/ DISTRIBUTION
- Variable oral absorption
- Undergoes first-pass metabolism
- Variable oral bioavailability 8–60%
- Protein binding < 20%

MOA
- Metabolised to α-methyl noradrenaline, which is an α_2 agonist
- This is taken up into nerve terminals in CNS, and when released decreases sympathetic tone

METABOLISM AND EXCRETION
- Hepatic metabolism
- Excreted in urine, 50% unchanged

METHYLDOPA
Phenylalanine derivative
Antihypertensive
- Tablets: 125/250/500 mg
- Solution: 50 mg/mL

DOSE
- 0.5–3 g/day in 2–3 doses

CHEMICAL PROPERTIES
- Nil

EFFECTS
CVS
- ↓ SVR and BP
- Postural hypotension (rare)
- Rebound hypertension if stopped suddenly

CNS
- Sedation
- Vertigo
- Depression, nightmares (uncommon)

RENAL
- Urine darkens on standing due to oxidation of methyldopa and its metabolites

GI
- Constipation
- Impaired liver function with long-term use
- Hepatic necrosis reported

HAEMATOLOGICAL
- Direct Coombe's test + in 10–20%
- Haemolytic anaemia
- Thrombocytopenia (rare)
- Leucopenia (rare)

OTHER
- Decreases MAC
- Hypersensitivity to drug can cause myocarditis
- Gynaecomastia

PRAZOSIN

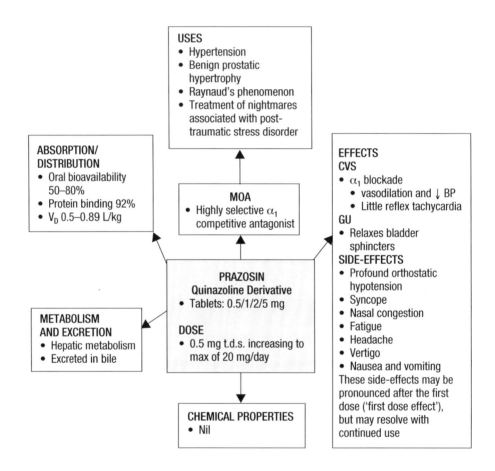

USES
- Hypertension
- Benign prostatic hypertrophy
- Raynaud's phenomenon
- Treatment of nightmares associated with post-traumatic stress disorder

ABSORPTION/ DISTRIBUTION
- Oral bioavailability 50–80%
- Protein binding 92%
- V_D 0.5–0.89 L/kg

MOA
- Highly selective α_1 competitive antagonist

EFFECTS
CVS
- α_1 blockade
  - vasodilation and ↓ BP
  - Little reflex tachycardia
GU
- Relaxes bladder sphincters
SIDE-EFFECTS
- Profound orthostatic hypotension
- Syncope
- Nasal congestion
- Fatigue
- Headache
- Vertigo
- Nausea and vomiting
These side-effects may be pronounced after the first dose ('first dose effect'), but may resolve with continued use

PRAZOSIN
Quinazoline Derivative
- Tablets: 0.5/1/2/5 mg

DOSE
- 0.5 mg t.d.s. increasing to max of 20 mg/day

METABOLISM AND EXCRETION
- Hepatic metabolism
- Excreted in bile

CHEMICAL PROPERTIES
- Nil

PHENOXYBENZAMINE

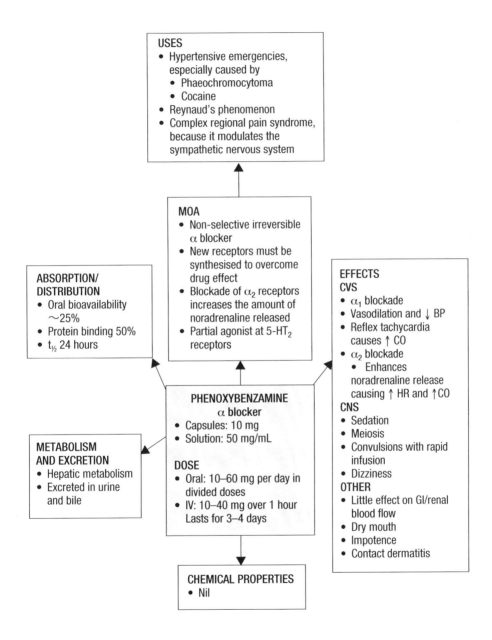

USES
- Hypertensive emergencies, especially caused by
  - Phaeochromocytoma
  - Cocaine
- Reynaud's phenomenon
- Complex regional pain syndrome, because it modulates the sympathetic nervous system

MOA
- Non-selective irreversible α blocker
- New receptors must be synthesised to overcome drug effect
- Blockade of α_2 receptors increases the amount of noradrenaline released
- Partial agonist at 5-HT_2 receptors

ABSORPTION/ DISTRIBUTION
- Oral bioavailability ~25%
- Protein binding 50%
- $t_{1/2}$ 24 hours

PHENOXYBENZAMINE
α **blocker**
- Capsules: 10 mg
- Solution: 50 mg/mL

DOSE
- Oral: 10–60 mg per day in divided doses
- IV: 10–40 mg over 1 hour Lasts for 3–4 days

METABOLISM AND EXCRETION
- Hepatic metabolism
- Excreted in urine and bile

EFFECTS
CVS
- α_1 blockade
- Vasodilation and ↓ BP
- Reflex tachycardia causes ↑ CO
- α_2 blockade
  - Enhances noradrenaline release causing ↑ HR and ↑CO

CNS
- Sedation
- Meiosis
- Convulsions with rapid infusion
- Dizziness

OTHER
- Little effect on GI/renal blood flow
- Dry mouth
- Impotence
- Contact dermatitis

CHEMICAL PROPERTIES
- Nil

PHENTOLAMINE

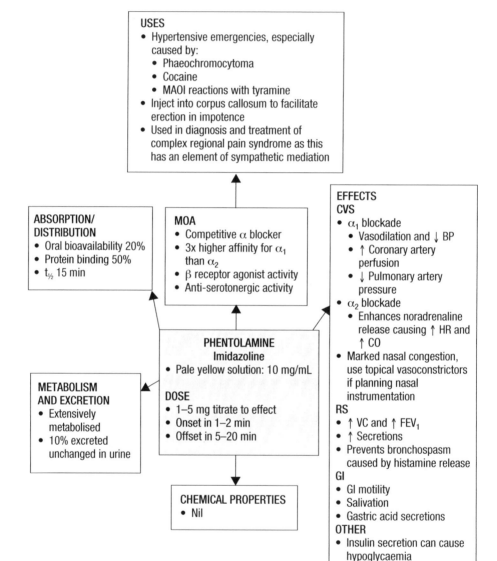

USES
- Hypertensive emergencies, especially caused by:
  - Phaeochromocytoma
  - Cocaine
  - MAOI reactions with tyramine
- Inject into corpus callosum to facilitate erection in impotence
- Used in diagnosis and treatment of complex regional pain syndrome as this has an element of sympathetic mediation

ABSORPTION/ DISTRIBUTION
- Oral bioavailability 20%
- Protein binding 50%
- $t_{1/2}$ 15 min

MOA
- Competitive α blocker
- 3x higher affinity for α_1 than α_2
- β receptor agonist activity
- Anti-serotonergic activity

EFFECTS
CVS
- α_1 blockade
  - Vasodilation and ↓ BP
  - ↑ Coronary artery perfusion
  - ↓ Pulmonary artery pressure
- α_2 blockade
  - Enhances noradrenaline release causing ↑ HR and ↑ CO
- Marked nasal congestion, use topical vasoconstrictors if planning nasal instrumentation

RS
- ↑ VC and ↑ FEV_1
- ↑ Secretions
- Prevents bronchospasm caused by histamine release

GI
- GI motility
- Salivation
- Gastric acid secretions

OTHER
- Insulin secretion can cause hypoglycaemia

PHENTOLAMINE
Imidazoline
- Pale yellow solution: 10 mg/mL

DOSE
- 1–5 mg titrate to effect
- Onset in 1–2 min
- Offset in 5–20 min

METABOLISM AND EXCRETION
- Extensively metabolised
- 10% excreted unchanged in urine

CHEMICAL PROPERTIES
- Nil

β BLOCKERS

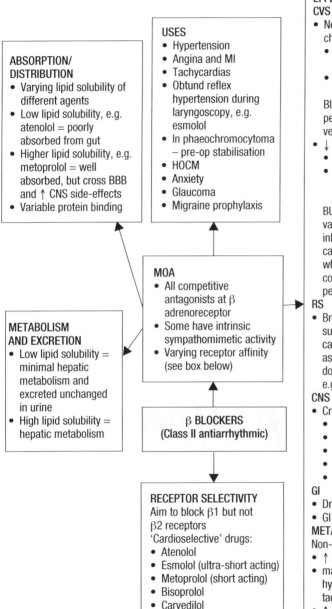

ABSORPTION/DISTRIBUTION
- Varying lipid solubility of different agents
- Low lipid solubility, e.g. atenolol = poorly absorbed from gut
- Higher lipid solubility, e.g. metoprolol = well absorbed, but cross BBB and ↑ CNS side-effects
- Variable protein binding

USES
- Hypertension
- Angina and MI
- Tachycardias
- Obtund reflex hypertension during laryngoscopy, e.g. esmolol
- In phaeochromocytoma – pre-op stabilisation
- HOCM
- Anxiety
- Glaucoma
- Migraine prophylaxis

MOA
- All competitive antagonists at β adrenoreceptor
- Some have intrinsic sympathomimetic activity
- Varying receptor affinity (see box below)

METABOLISM AND EXCRETION
- Low lipid solubility = minimal hepatic metabolism and excreted unchanged in urine
- High lipid solubility = hepatic metabolism

β BLOCKERS (Class II antiarrhythmic)

RECEPTOR SELECTIVITY
Aim to block β1 but not β2 receptors
'Cardioselective' drugs:
- Atenolol
- Esmolol (ultra-short acting)
- Metoprolol (short acting)
- Bisoprolol
- Carvedilol

NB all will act on β2 if dose high enough

EFFECTS
CVS
- Negative ionotrope and chronotrope so:
  - ↑ Time in diastole and ↑ coronary artery perfusion
  - ↓ Cardiac oxygen requirements
  BUT, may worsen performance of failing ventricle
- ↓ BP
  - ↓ HR and CO
  - ↓ Renin secretion by β_1 inhibition at juxtaglomerular apparatus
  BUT: beware in peripheral vascular disease as inhibition of β_2 receptors causes some constriction which may further compromise circulation in peripheries

RS
- Bronchospasm, worse in susceptible patients so give cardioselective drugs in asthma/COPD and give test dose of short acting drug, e.g. esmolol/metoprolol

CNS
- Cross BBB can cause:
  - Hallucinations
  - Nightmares
  - Depression
  - Fatigue
  - ↓ Intraocular pressure

GI
- Dry mouth
- GI upset

METABOLIC
Non-selective agents can:
- ↑ Resting BM in diabetics
- mask symptoms of hypoglycaemia (sweating, tachycardia, etc)
- ↑ Triglycerides and ↓ HDL

CHAPTER 26

Diuretics

Draw a nephron and indicate where diuretic drugs exert their effects

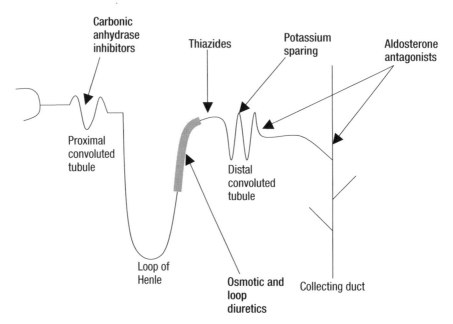

FIGURE 1.35 Schematic representation of the nephron indicating the sites of action of various diuretic agents

How does mannitol exert its effects?
➤ Mannitol is a sugar alcohol solution, which works as an osmotic diuretic.
➤ The drug has a molecular weight of 182 Daltons and so is freely filtered by the glomerulus, but not reabsorbed.
➤ It increases the osmolality of the filtrate and so water follows the drug to be excreted.

What is the major indication for using mannitol?
Mannitol is used primarily in the treatment of raised intracerebral pressure (ICP). It reduces ICP by:
➤ Decreasing the formation of CSF.
➤ Decreasing plasma volume and thereby encouraging water to move out of the brain, reducing oedema. Mannitol does not cross the intact blood brain barrier. However, if the membrane is disrupted, mannitol can cross it and worsen oedema by drawing water with it. Hence, unless a patient is actively coning, it should only be used on the advice of a neurosurgeon.
➤ It is free radical scavenger and so may afford some additional neuroprotection.

Can mannitol be used repeatedly?
No, mannitol is used to 'buy time' until raised ICP can be treated definitively. The dose cannot be repeated indefinitely, as it will cause an unacceptable rise in serum osmolality and circulatory overload. With repeated dosing it will eventually cross the blood brain barrier and cause a rise in ICP.

What are the side-effects of the thiazides and loop diuretics?
Please refer to the appropriate spider diagram for this answer.

How are diuretics used in renal failure?
Diuretics do not reverse renal failure, but they can be used to control its symptoms. The use of diuretics, particularly loop diuretics, reduces:
➤ hypertension, mediated by decreased sodium excretion and water retention
➤ congestive cardiac failure caused by circulatory overload
➤ oedema.

Large doses of the drugs may be needed as their efficacy is decreased in the face of low renal blood flow, reducing delivery to their target organ. It may be necessary to give the drugs by continuous infusion and to combine various diuretics to achieve optimum results.

LOOP DIURETICS

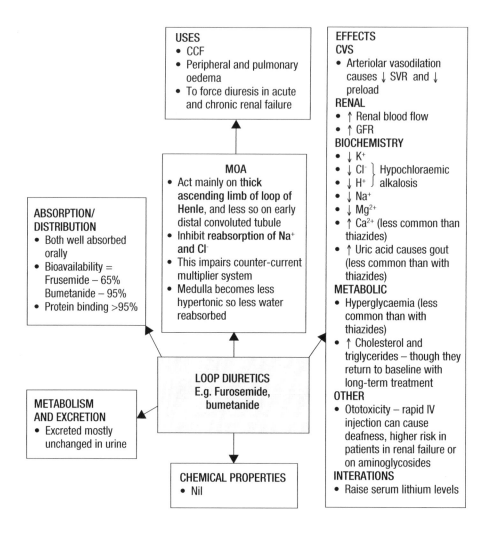

USES
- CCF
- Peripheral and pulmonary oedema
- To force diuresis in acute and chronic renal failure

MOA
- Act mainly on **thick ascending limb of loop of Henle,** and less so on early distal convoluted tubule
- Inhibit **reabsorption of Na^+ and Cl^-**
- This impairs counter-current multiplier system
- Medulla becomes less hypertonic so less water reabsorbed

ABSORPTION/ DISTRIBUTION
- Both well absorbed orally
- Bioavailability = Frusemide – 65% Bumetanide – 95%
- Protein binding >95%

METABOLISM AND EXCRETION
- Excreted mostly unchanged in urine

LOOP DIURETICS E.g. Furosemide, bumetanide

CHEMICAL PROPERTIES
- Nil

EFFECTS
CVS
- Arteriolar vasodilation causes ↓ SVR and ↓ preload

RENAL
- ↑ Renal blood flow
- ↑ GFR

BIOCHEMISTRY
- ↓ K^+
- ↓ Cl^- } Hypochloraemic
- ↓ H^+ } alkalosis
- ↓ Na^+
- ↓ Mg^{2+}
- ↑ Ca^{2+} (less common than thiazides)
- ↑ Uric acid causes gout (less common than with thiazides)

METABOLIC
- Hyperglycaemia (less common than with thiazides)
- ↑ Cholesterol and triglycerides – though they return to baseline with long-term treatment

OTHER
- Ototoxicity – rapid IV injection can cause deafness, higher risk in patients in renal failure or on aminoglycosides

INTERATIONS
- Raise serum lithium levels

THIAZIDE DIURETICS

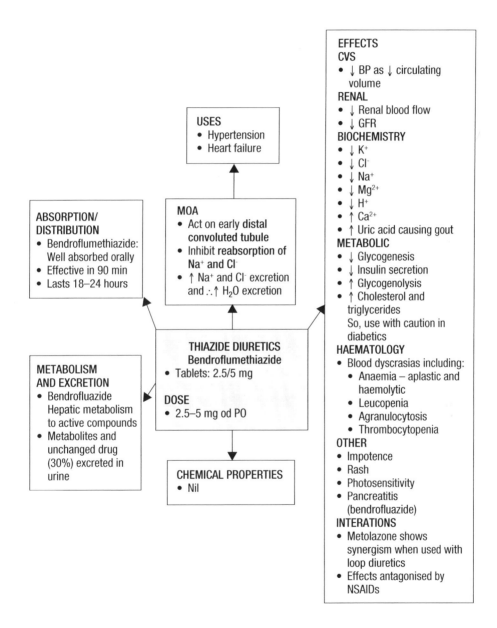

USES
- Hypertension
- Heart failure

ABSORPTION/ DISTRIBUTION
- Bendroflumethiazide: Well absorbed orally
- Effective in 90 min
- Lasts 18–24 hours

MOA
- Act on early **distal convoluted tubule**
- Inhibit **reabsorption of** Na^+ and Cl^-
- $\uparrow$ Na^+ and Cl^- excretion and $\therefore \uparrow$ H_2O excretion

METABOLISM AND EXCRETION
- Bendrofluazide Hepatic metabolism to active compounds
- Metabolites and unchanged drug (30%) excreted in urine

THIAZIDE DIURETICS
Bendroflumethiazide
- Tablets: 2.5/5 mg

DOSE
- 2.5–5 mg od PO

CHEMICAL PROPERTIES
- Nil

EFFECTS
CVS
- $\downarrow$ BP as $\downarrow$ circulating volume

RENAL
- $\downarrow$ Renal blood flow
- $\downarrow$ GFR

BIOCHEMISTRY
- $\downarrow$ K^+
- $\downarrow$ Cl^-
- $\downarrow$ Na^+
- $\downarrow$ Mg^{2+}
- $\downarrow$ H^+
- $\uparrow$ Ca^{2+}
- $\uparrow$ Uric acid causing gout

METABOLIC
- $\downarrow$ Glycogenesis
- $\downarrow$ Insulin secretion
- $\uparrow$ Glycogenolysis
- $\uparrow$ Cholesterol and triglycerides
So, use with caution in diabetics

HAEMATOLOGY
- Blood dyscrasias including:
  - Anaemia – aplastic and haemolytic
  - Leucopenia
  - Agranulocytosis
  - Thrombocytopenia

OTHER
- Impotence
- Rash
- Photosensitivity
- Pancreatitis (bendrofluazide)

INTERATIONS
- Metolazone shows synergism when used with loop diuretics
- Effects antagonised by NSAIDs

K⁺ SPARING DIURETICS

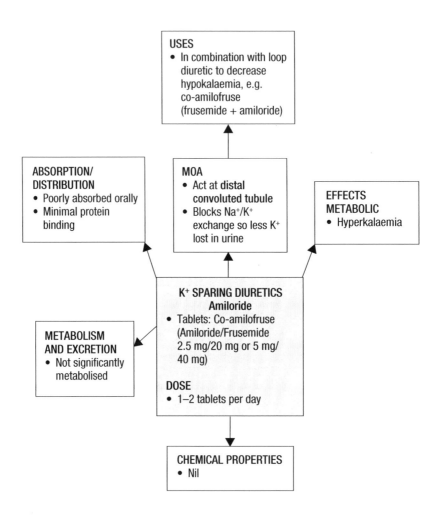

USES
- In combination with loop diuretic to decrease hypokalaemia, e.g. co-amilofruse (frusemide + amiloride)

ABSORPTION/ DISTRIBUTION
- Poorly absorbed orally
- Minimal protein binding

MOA
- Act at distal convoluted tubule
- Blocks Na⁺/K⁺ exchange so less K⁺ lost in urine

EFFECTS METABOLIC
- Hyperkalaemia

K⁺ SPARING DIURETICS
Amiloride
- Tablets: Co-amilofruse (Amiloride/Frusemide 2.5 mg/20 mg or 5 mg/ 40 mg)

DOSE
- 1–2 tablets per day

METABOLISM AND EXCRETION
- Not significantly metabolised

CHEMICAL PROPERTIES
- Nil

SPIRONOLACTONE

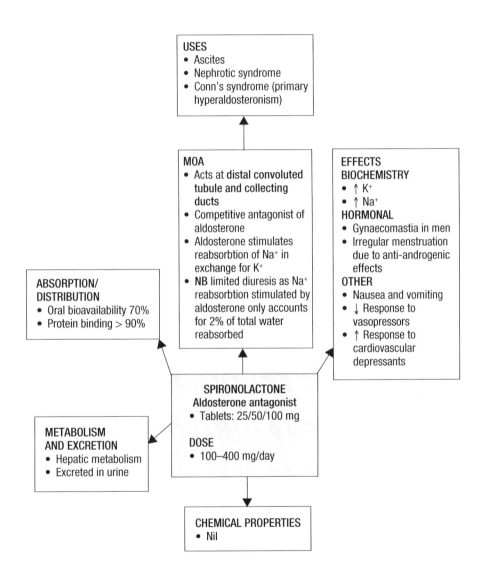

USES
- Ascites
- Nephrotic syndrome
- Conn's syndrome (primary hyperaldosteronism)

MOA
- Acts at distal convoluted tubule and collecting ducts
- Competitive antagonist of aldosterone
- Aldosterone stimulates reabsorbtion of Na$^+$ in exchange for K$^+$
- **NB** limited diuresis as Na$^+$ reabsorbtion stimulated by aldosterone only accounts for 2% of total water reabsorbed

EFFECTS
BIOCHEMISTRY
- ↑ K$^+$
- ↑ Na$^+$
HORMONAL
- Gynaecomastia in men
- Irregular menstruation due to anti-androgenic effects
OTHER
- Nausea and vomiting
- ↓ Response to vasopressors
- ↑ Response to cardiovascular depressants

ABSORPTION/ DISTRIBUTION
- Oral bioavailability 70%
- Protein binding > 90%

SPIRONOLACTONE
Aldosterone antagonist
- Tablets: 25/50/100 mg

DOSE
- 100–400 mg/day

METABOLISM AND EXCRETION
- Hepatic metabolism
- Excreted in urine

CHEMICAL PROPERTIES
- Nil

ACETAZOLAMIDE

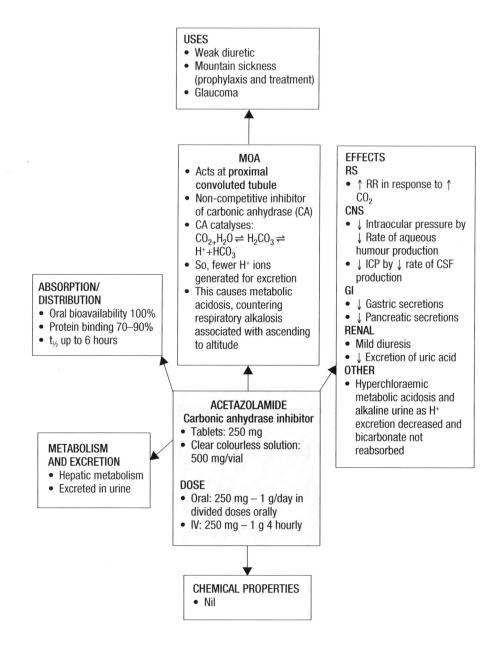

USES
- Weak diuretic
- Mountain sickness (prophylaxis and treatment)
- Glaucoma

MOA
- Acts at **proximal convoluted tubule**
- Non-competitive inhibitor of carbonic anhydrase (CA)
- CA catalyses: $CO_2 + H_2O \rightleftharpoons H_2CO_3 \rightleftharpoons H^+ + HCO_3^-$
- So, fewer H^+ ions generated for excretion
- This causes metabolic acidosis, countering respiratory alkalosis associated with ascending to altitude

EFFECTS
RS
- ↑ RR in response to ↑ CO_2

CNS
- ↓ Intraocular pressure by ↓ Rate of aqueous humour production
- ↓ ICP by ↓ rate of CSF production

GI
- ↓ Gastric secretions
- ↓ Pancreatic secretions

RENAL
- Mild diuresis
- ↓ Excretion of uric acid

OTHER
- Hyperchloraemic metabolic acidosis and alkaline urine as H^+ excretion decreased and bicarbonate not reabsorbed

ABSORPTION/ DISTRIBUTION
- Oral bioavailability 100%
- Protein binding 70–90%
- $t_{1/2}$ up to 6 hours

ACETAZOLAMIDE
Carbonic anhydrase inhibitor
- Tablets: 250 mg
- Clear colourless solution: 500 mg/vial

DOSE
- Oral: 250 mg – 1 g/day in divided doses orally
- IV: 250 mg – 1 g 4 hourly

METABOLISM AND EXCRETION
- Hepatic metabolism
- Excreted in urine

CHEMICAL PROPERTIES
- Nil

MANNITOL

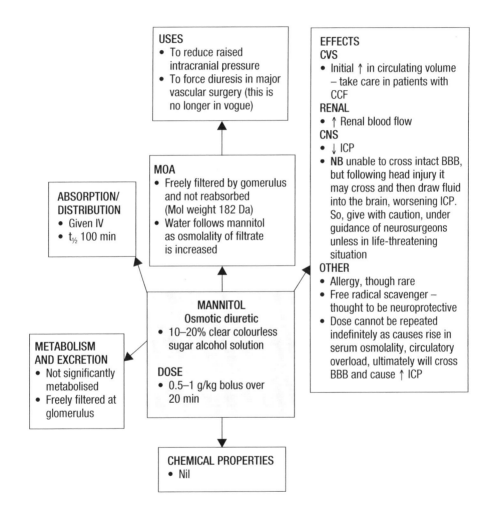

USES
- To reduce raised intracranial pressure
- To force diuresis in major vascular surgery (this is no longer in vogue)

EFFECTS
CVS
- Initial ↑ in circulating volume – take care in patients with CCF

RENAL
- ↑ Renal blood flow

CNS
- ↓ ICP
- **NB** unable to cross intact BBB, but following head injury it may cross and then draw fluid into the brain, worsening ICP. So, give with caution, under guidance of neurosurgeons unless in life-threatening situation

OTHER
- Allergy, though rare
- Free radical scavenger – thought to be neuroprotective
- Dose cannot be repeated indefinitely as causes rise in serum osmality, circulatory overload, ultimately will cross BBB and cause ↑ ICP

MOA
- Freely filtered by gomerulus and not reabsorbed (Mol weight 182 Da)
- Water follows mannitol as osmolality of filtrate is increased

ABSORPTION/ DISTRIBUTION
- Given IV
- $t_{1/2}$ 100 min

METABOLISM AND EXCRETION
- Not significantly metabolised
- Freely filtered at glomerulus

MANNITOL
Osmotic diuretic
- 10–20% clear colourless sugar alcohol solution

DOSE
- 0.5–1 g/kg bolus over 20 min

CHEMICAL PROPERTIES
- Nil

CHAPTER 27

Non-steroidal anti-inflammatory drugs

How do NSAIDs exert their effects?

NSAIDs exert their effects by inhibiting the action of the enzyme cyclo-oxygenase (COX) and therefore reducing the production of the inflammatory prostanoids, as shown below:

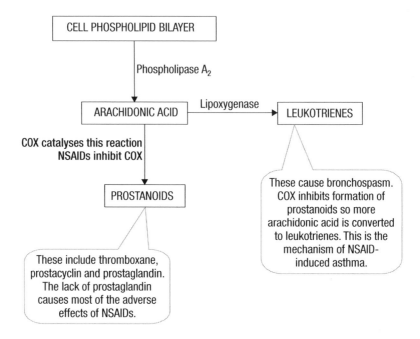

FIGURE 1.36 Pathway for prostaglandin and leukotriene synthesis

Describe the distribution of cyclo-oxygenase

There are two types of COX when discussing NSAIDs: COX 1 and COX 2.

➤ **COX 1** (constitutive) is found in most cells.
➤ **COX 2** (inducible) is undetectable in most normal tissue but found in abundance in macrophages and other cells of inflammation.
  ● COX 2 catalyses the formation of inflammatory mediators and is therefore the enzyme that needs to be inhibited in order to decrease pain and inflammation. In theory, if COX 2 could be inhibited without affecting COX 1, symptoms would be improved with minimal or no side-effects. In practice, this is not the case as COX 2 inhibitors still show the side-effect profile of non-specific agents.

What are the main actions of prostacyclin and thromboxane?

➤ **Prostacyclin** is a vasodilator and prevents formation of platelet plug in primary haemostasis.

➤ **Thromboxane** is produced by platelets. It is a vasoconstrictor and a potent platelet aggregator.

These prostanoids are in fine balance in health.

Describe the main actions of prostaglandins

Prostaglandins – nine different receptors result in varied actions, e.g.:
➤ PGE_2 – ↓ gastric acid secretion ↑ gastric mucous secretion
➤ PGI_2 – vasodilatation, platelet aggregation
➤ $PGF_{2\alpha}$ – uterine contraction, bronchoconstriction.

Classify the NSAIDs

➤ NSAIDs may be classified according to their structure:
  • salicylic acids, e.g. aspirin (acetylsalicylic acid)
  • phenylacetic acids, e.g. diclofenac
  • carboacetic acids, e.g. indomethacin
  • proprionic acids, e.g. ibuprofen
  • enolic acids, e.g. piroxicam
➤ NSAIDs may also be classified according to their inhibition of cyclo-oxygenase: non-specific versus selective COX 2:
  • non-selective COX inhibitors, e.g. aspirin, diclofenac, ibuprofen
  • COX 2 inhibitors, e.g. parecoxib.

What are the indications for use of NSAIDs?

NSAIDs are used therapeutically for their anti-inflammatory and analgesic effects. In the management of acute pain, NSAIDs have an opioid sparing effect.

Aspirin compared to the other NSAIDs has a unique anti-platelet action, which is used therapeutically in the prevention of arterial thrombosis (myocardial infarction and cerebrovascular accident).

What are the main contraindications to the use of NSAIDs?

➤ Relative contraindications to NSAIDs include renal impairment, history of gastrointestinal bleeding, heart failure, hypertension, coagulation defects.
➤ Absolute contraindications include proven hypersensitivity to aspirin or any NSAIDs.
➤ Assess the hydration status of the patient before prescribing NSAIDs. There is a risk of precipitating renal failure if NSAIDs are administered to patients who are dehydrated.
➤ NSAIDs may enhance the effects of warfarin.
➤ NSAIDs may worsen asthma in 10–20% of patients; they are contraindicated if aspirin or any other NSAIDs has precipitated attacks of asthma, although this occurs rarely in children.
➤ Aspirin should not be given to children under 12 years for analgesia or children under 15 years as an antipyretic because of the risk of Reye's syndrome (aspirin-induced liver failure secondary to mitochondrial dysfunction).

What are the main side-effects of NSAIDs?

The more a NSAID blocks COX 1, the greater is its tendency to cause peptic ulceration and promote bleeding. Selective COX 2 inhibitors cause less bleeding and fewer ulcers than other NSAIDs but certain drugs in this group have been associated with an increased incidence of thrombotic complications, especially myocardial infarction (rofecoxib was withdrawn in 2004 because of an increased incidence of myocardial infarction).

The following list summarises the main side-effects of NSAIDs:
➤ NSAIDs-induced exacerbation of asthma (approximately 10–20% of asthmatics

affected). The mechanism is thought to involve increased production of bronchoconstricting leukotrienes.

➤ Gastrointestinal bleeding – NSAIDs reduce circulating prostaglandins which are essential in maintaining gastric mucosal integrity.

➤ Acute kidney injury may be induced by NSAIDs in vulnerable patients, e.g. pre-existing renal dysfunction, diabetics, elderly or dehydrated patients. The mechanism involves reduced levels of prostacyclin, which are required to maintain renal perfusion.

➤ Platelet dysfunction – related to reduced thromboxane production. This is seen only with the non-specific COX inhibitors, not with the selective COX 2 inhibitors.

PARACETAMOL

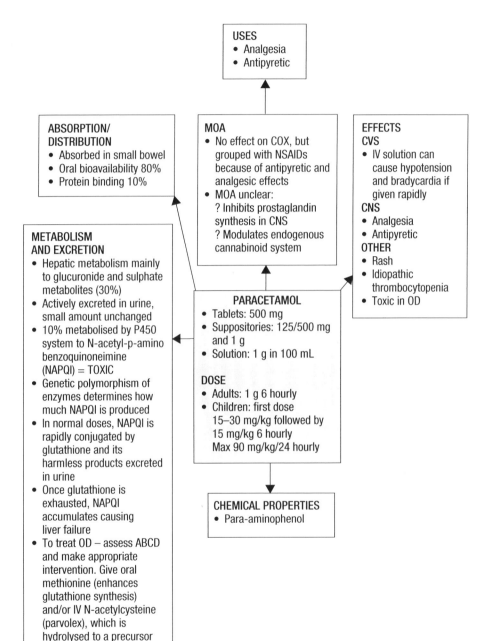

USES
- Analgesia
- Antipyretic

ABSORPTION/ DISTRIBUTION
- Absorbed in small bowel
- Oral bioavailability 80%
- Protein binding 10%

MOA
- No effect on COX, but grouped with NSAIDs because of antipyretic and analgesic effects
- MOA unclear:
  ? Inhibits prostaglandin synthesis in CNS
  ? Modulates endogenous cannabinoid system

EFFECTS
CVS
- IV solution can cause hypotension and bradycardia if given rapidly
CNS
- Analgesia
- Antipyretic
OTHER
- Rash
- Idiopathic thrombocytopenia
- Toxic in OD

METABOLISM AND EXCRETION
- Hepatic metabolism mainly to glucuronide and sulphate metabolites (30%)
- Actively excreted in urine, small amount unchanged
- 10% metabolised by P450 system to N-acetyl-p-amino benzoquinoneimine (NAPQI) = TOXIC
- Genetic polymorphism of enzymes determines how much NAPQI is produced
- In normal doses, NAPQI is rapidly conjugated by glutathione and its harmless products excreted in urine
- Once glutathione is exhausted, NAPQI accumulates causing liver failure
- To treat OD – assess ABCD and make appropriate intervention. Give oral methionine (enhances glutathione synthesis) and/or IV N-acetylcysteine (parvolex), which is hydrolysed to a precursor of glutathione

PARACETAMOL
- Tablets: 500 mg
- Suppositories: 125/500 mg and 1 g
- Solution: 1 g in 100 mL

DOSE
- Adults: 1 g 6 hourly
- Children: first dose 15–30 mg/kg followed by 15 mg/kg 6 hourly Max 90 mg/kg/24 hourly

CHEMICAL PROPERTIES
- Para-aminophenol

ASPIRIN

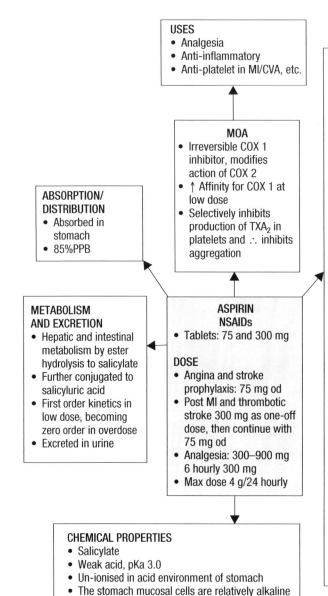

USES
- Analgesia
- Anti-inflammatory
- Anti-platelet in MI/CVA, etc.

MOA
- Irreversible COX 1 inhibitor, modifies action of COX 2
- ↑ Affinity for COX 1 at low dose
- Selectively inhibits production of TXA$_2$ in platelets and ∴ inhibits aggregation

ABSORPTION/ DISTRIBUTION
- Absorbed in stomach
- 85%PPB

METABOLISM AND EXCRETION
- Hepatic and intestinal metabolism by ester hydrolysis to salicylate
- Further conjugated to salicyluric acid
- First order kinetics in low dose, becoming zero order in overdose
- Excreted in urine

ASPIRIN
NSAIDs
- Tablets: 75 and 300 mg

DOSE
- Angina and stroke prophylaxis: 75 mg od
- Post MI and thrombotic stroke 300 mg as one-off dose, then continue with 75 mg od
- Analgesia: 300–900 mg 6 hourly 300 mg
- Max dose 4 g/24 hourly

EFFECTS
RS
- 20% of asthmatics sensitive to NSAIDs which can cause bronchoconstriction
GI
- ↑ Risk of GI bleeding and ulceration because inhibition of prostaglandin (PG) synthesis causes ↓ mucosal protection
- Hepatotoxic causing transaminitis
RENAL
- Inhibition of PGs and prostacyclin causes local hypoxia and ↓ renal perfusion
CVS
- ↓ Endoperoxidases and thromboxane A$_2$ ∴ ↓ platelet aggregation and ↓ vasoconstriction, ∴ cardioprotective
- NB effects on platelet irreversible. New platelets must be synthesised to reverse effect
- Fluid retention can precipitate heart failure
DRUG INTERACTIONS
- Care with warfarin – NSAIDs are highly protein bound and so may displace warfarin
- May ↑ lithium levels
OTHER
- Toxic in overdose
- Reye's syndrome in children

CHEMICAL PROPERTIES
- Salicylate
- Weak acid, pKa 3.0
- Un-ionised in acid environment of stomach
- The stomach mucosal cells are relatively alkaline and so salicylate can become ionised and trapped in cells ∴ unable to reach circulation

DICLOFENAC

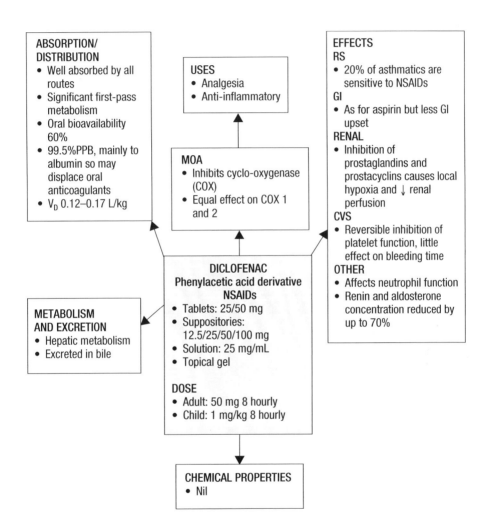

ABSORPTION/ DISTRIBUTION
- Well absorbed by all routes
- Significant first-pass metabolism
- Oral bioavailability 60%
- 99.5%PPB, mainly to albumin so may displace oral anticoagulants
- V_D 0.12–0.17 L/kg

USES
- Analgesia
- Anti-inflammatory

MOA
- Inhibits cyclo-oxygenase (COX)
- Equal effect on COX 1 and 2

EFFECTS
RS
- 20% of asthmatics are sensitive to NSAIDs
GI
- As for aspirin but less GI upset
RENAL
- Inhibition of prostaglandins and prostacyclins causes local hypoxia and ↓ renal perfusion
CVS
- Reversible inhibition of platelet function, little effect on bleeding time
OTHER
- Affects neutrophil function
- Renin and aldosterone concentration reduced by up to 70%

METABOLISM AND EXCRETION
- Hepatic metabolism
- Excreted in bile

DICLOFENAC
Phenylacetic acid derivative NSAIDs
- Tablets: 25/50 mg
- Suppositories: 12.5/25/50/100 mg
- Solution: 25 mg/mL
- Topical gel

DOSE
- Adult: 50 mg 8 hourly
- Child: 1 mg/kg 8 hourly

CHEMICAL PROPERTIES
- Nil

CHAPTER 28

Antibiotics

How do antibiotics exert their effects?

Antibiotics are drugs used to inhibit (bacteriostatic) or kill (bacteriocidal) bacteria. Their mode of action can be classified as shown in Figure 1.37.

Which factors should be considered when administering gentamicin?

➤ Aminoglycoside antibiotics such as gentamicin are used to treat urinary and biliary tract infections, endocarditis and septicaemia.

➤ They work by binding irreversibly to the 30S subunit of the bacterial ribosome and inhibiting bacterial protein synthesis. This leads to bacterial cell death.

➤ These agents are administered intravenously or intramuscularly, as they are not absorbed enterally.

➤ At high plasma concentrations aminoglycosides can cause ototoxicity and nephrotoxicity.

➤ The dose of gentamicin is 3–5 mg/kg/day and can be given in divided doses every 8 hours. Blood samples are taken 1 hour after the administered dose ('peak' plasma concentration) and/or just before a dose ('trough' plasma concentration). 'Peak' plasma gentamicin levels should be 5–10 mg/L and 'trough' levels should be less than 2 mg/L.

➤ An alternative, once-daily regime is used in some departments. Here, the full gentamicin dose is prescribed as a single dose and the frequency of administration is adjusted according to the 'trough' gentamicin levels using a nomogram, e.g. the Urban Craig nomogram.

In which patient groups should gentamicin be used with caution?

➤ Gentamicin should be used with caution during pregnancy as it can cross the placenta and cause fetal ototoxicity.

➤ Aminoglycosides are not metabolised, instead they are excreted unchanged by the kidneys, primarily by glomerular filtration. Therefore the dose and/or frequency of administration should be altered in renal failure. Renal function should be quantified using the creatinine clearance, which can be estimated using the Cockcroft and Gault formula.

➤ Aminoglycosides can potentiate the action of non-depolarising muscle relaxants or cause recurrence of the blockade produced by these agents. They cause this effect by interfering with calcium entry into the presynaptic terminal of the motor axon, thereby preventing the release of acetylcholine from the presynaptic vesicles. This drug interaction can even cause a neostigmine-resistant block, which can be antagonised by the use of calcium salts. Because of this effect on neurotransmission, aminoglycosides are contraindicated in patients with myasthenia gravis.

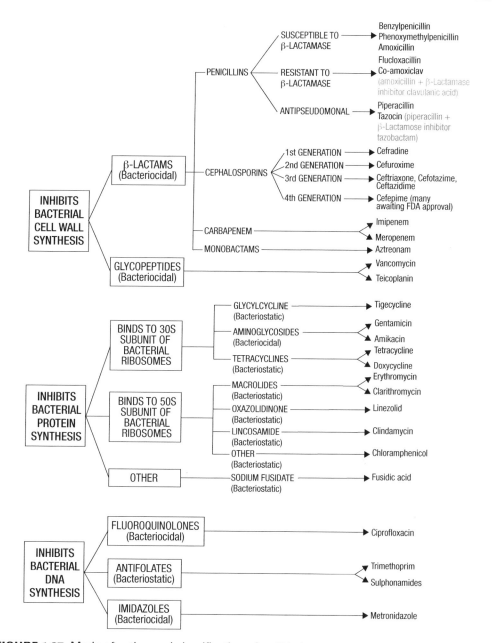

FIGURE 1.37 Mode of action and classification of antibiotics

Cockcroft and Gault formula to estimate creatinine clearance (CrCl):

$$\text{CrCl in men} = \frac{1.23\,(140\ \text{age in years})\ \text{weight in kg}}{\text{Serum creatinine}\ (\mu\text{mol/L})}$$

$$\text{CrCl in females} = \frac{1.04\,(140\ \text{age in years})\ \text{weight in kg}}{\text{Serum creatinine}\ (\mu\text{mol/L})}$$

Describe the structure of penicillin
➤ The basic structure comprises a thiazolidine ring nucleus attached to a β-lactam ring.
➤ The β-lactam ring has an amino-acid side chain, which varies between different types of penicillin, and determines their main antibacterial and pharmacological properties.
➤ Other antimicrobial agents belonging the β-lactam group of antibiotics include:
  ● cephalosporins
  ● monobactams
  ● carbapenems.

Describe the mechanism of action of penicillin
➤ Penicillins are bactericidal antibiotics that inhibit bacterial cell wall synthesis.
➤ The β-lactam ring binds to bacterial cell wall proteins and inhibits the formation of peptidoglycan cross-links. These cross-links are essential for maintaining bacterial cell wall stability and without them the wall is weakened, resulting in cytolysis and cell death due to osmotic pressures.
➤ The resultant build-up of peptidoglycan precursors stimulates the bacterial release of enzymes, which auto-digest the bacterial cell wall.

What is their spectrum of clinical use?
➤ Penicillins are active against most Gram-positive organisms and some Gram-negative cocci.
➤ They are not very effective against Gram-negative bacilli.
➤ Penicillins can be divided into categories depending on their spectrum of action:
  ● narrow spectrum, e.g. benzylpenicillin
  ● β-lactamase resistant, e.g. flucloxacillin
  ● broad spectrum, e.g. ampicillin
  ● anti-pseudomonal, e.g. piperacillin.

How does resistance to penicillins develop?
There are several mechanisms by which bacteria develop resistance to penicillins:
➤ **Drug inactivation** – bacterial production of β-lactamase leads to hydrolysis of the β-lactam ring.
➤ **Alteration of penicillin binding proteins** – this prevents the antibiotics from binding onto the bacterial cell wall.
➤ **Alteration of bacterial cell wall permeability** – this prevents antibiotics from penetrating the cell wall.

What are the major side-effects of the penicillins?
➤ **Hypersensitivity** due to an allergy to the basic structure of the β-lactam group of the antibiotics. Therefore, up to 10% of patients allergic to penicillin will suffer cross-reactivity if given another antibiotic containing a β-lactam group. Hypersensitivity reactions occur in 10% of the population while anaphylaxis occurs in approximately 0.01%.
➤ **Gastrointestinal disturbances.**
➤ **Encephalopathy** in patients with renal failure.
➤ **Rash**, especially when ampicillin is administered to patients with infectious mononucleosis.

How do penicillins and aminoglycosides act synergistically?
Penicillins weaken the bacterial cell wall by inhibiting cell wall synthesis and this enables the aminoglycosides to penetrate the cell and inhibit bacterial protein synthesis intracellularly.

CHAPTER 29

Anticoagulants

What types of heparin do you know?

Naturally occurring heparin
➤ A highly sulphated glycosaminoglycan carbohydrate weighing between 3000 and 50 000 Daltons.
➤ It is produced by basophils and mast cells.

Unfractionated heparin (UFH)
➤ Synthetic agent weighing between 5000 and 25 000 Daltons.
➤ It binds to and potentiates the action of antithrombin III 1000-fold.
➤ Activated antithrombin III inhibits thrombin and other serine proteases that promote blood clotting.

Low molecular weight heparin (LMWH), e.g. enoxaparin, dalteparin, tinzaparin
➤ More recently developed drugs weighing between 2000 and 8000 Daltons.
➤ LMWHs do not target antithrombin, but instead directly inhibit factor Xa.

The dose of both LMWH and UFH are calculated in units of activity rather than weight. One unit of activity is the amount of a preparation required to keep 1 mL of cat's blood fluid for 24 hours at 0°C.

Figure 1.38 shows the final common pathway of clotting.

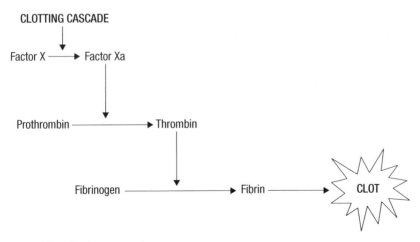

FIGURE 1.38 The clotting cascade

What are the differences between the unfractionated (UFH) and low molecular weight heparins (LMWH)?

In order to inactivate thrombin, the heparin molecule must be able to bind both the antithrombin III molecule and the thrombin molecule. To do this it must have a size greater than 18 saccharide ternary units. Smaller molecules, therefore, are only able to inhibit the activity of other proteases such as factor Xa.

TABLE 1.39 Comparison of unfractionated and low molecular weight heparins

	UFH	LMWH
Xa inhibition	+	+++
Protein binding	50%	10%
$t_{1/2}$	30–150 min (dose-dependent)	2–3x longer for equivalent dose
Monitoring	APTT	Anti-Xa
Administration	Monitored infusion	Once daily (or BD). Not routinely monitored
Bioavailability (sc dose)	40%	90%

How is heparin used clinically?
➤ **UFH:**
- As an infusion to prevent the propagation of deep vein thrombosis (DVT) and pulmonary emboli (PE).
- During cardiopulmonary bypass to reduce clotting of blood in contact with bypass circuit.
- During extracorporeal membrane oxygenation (ECMO) to prevent clotting in the circuit.
- During vascular surgery to prevent newly inserted stent occlusion.
- Twice daily subcutaneous dose for thrombosis prophylaxis.

Its half-life is only around 1 hour and so UFH must be given continuously by infusion. It is common practice to give a bolus of 5000 IU followed by an infusion based on the patient's weight. The patient's APTT is measured 6 hours following the start of the infusion, and the dose is adjusted to keep the APTT at 1.5–2x normal. Because of its short half-life, the anticoagulant effects of UFH are quickly lost once the infusion is stopped. This can prove useful, e.g. if bleeding becomes a problem, or if the patient needs to go to theatre.

➤ **LMWH:**
- As a twice daily subcutaneous injection to prevent the propagation of DVT and PE.
- As a twice daily subcutaneous injection to prevent clot propagation in acute coronary syndrome.
- Once daily subcutaneous dose for thrombosis prophylaxis.

Because of its longer half-life, LMWH can be given once or twice daily depending on the indication.

How is heparin therapy monitored?
Activated partial thromboplastin time (APTT) measures the activity of the intrinsic clotting cascade (factors VIII, XI, XI and XII) and the final common pathway and is therefore, prolonged by UFH. Hence, we measure APTT to monitor and alter heparin infusions appropriately.

LMWH inhibits mainly factor Xa and therefore does not affect the APTT. Usually no monitoring is required but anti-factor Xa levels can be measured as needed.

What are the side-effects of heparin therapy?
➤ **Haemorrhage:**
  • Heparin is given subcutaneously to avoid intramuscular haematoma. It can cause fatal haemorrhage if given in overdose. Its dose should be reduced in patients with renal failure, in whom it can accumulate. UFH, but not LMWH, can be reversed with protamine (dose 1 mg reverses 100 IU heparin)
➤ **Non-immune thrombocytopenia:**
  • Occurs after approximately 4 days of therapy.
  • Platelets recover spontaneously without cessation of heparin.
➤ **Heparin-induced thrombocytopenia (HIT):**
  • This immune-mediated process usually takes around 5 days to develop, though prior exposure to heparin can cause an accelerated course.
  • IgG antibodies are made against heparin after it binds to platelet factor 4 (PF4).
  • These antibodies attach themselves to the heparin PF4 complex and go on to bind and activate platelets. Consequently, thrombi are formed throughout the vascular tree and the platelet count falls. HIT can result in fatal PEs, limb ischaemia and stroke.
  • In suspected HIT heparin should be discontinued and blood sent to the lab for a 'HIT screen'. Alternative anticoagulation should be used.
➤ **Hypotension:**
  • Can follow rapid bolusing of a large dose.
➤ **Other:**
  • Osteoporosis following long-term administration.
  • Alopecia.

What are the advantages of LMWH?
➤ It only requires once or twice daily dosing.
➤ It does not need monitoring.
➤ It is less likely to cause HIT (though it can still do so) and non-immune mediated thrombocytopenia.

How does warfarin exert its anticoagulant effect?
Warfarin is primarily indicated in the treatment of deep vein thrombosis, atrial fibrillation in patients at risk of embolisation and patients with mechanical prosthetic heart valves. It exerts its anticoagulant effect by inhibiting the synthesis of the vitamin K dependent clotting factors (II, VII, IX and X). Anticoagulant effect is monitored via the international normalised ratio (INR).

Which class of drugs may alter the plasma protein binding of warfarin?
Warfarin is extensively protein bound (>95%). NSAIDs if administered concurrently with warfarin compete for the plasma protein binding sites, leading to warfarin displacement and increased warfarin anticoagulant effect.

Describe the treatment of overdose of warfarin
The main adverse effect of warfarin overdose is bleeding. Major bleeding should be managed using an 'ABC' approach. Specific treatment includes stopping the warfarin, administration of vitamin K (10 mg IV), administration of dried prothrombin complex (which contain factors II, VII, IX and X) or alternatively administration of 15 mL/kg of fresh frozen plasma.

HEPARIN

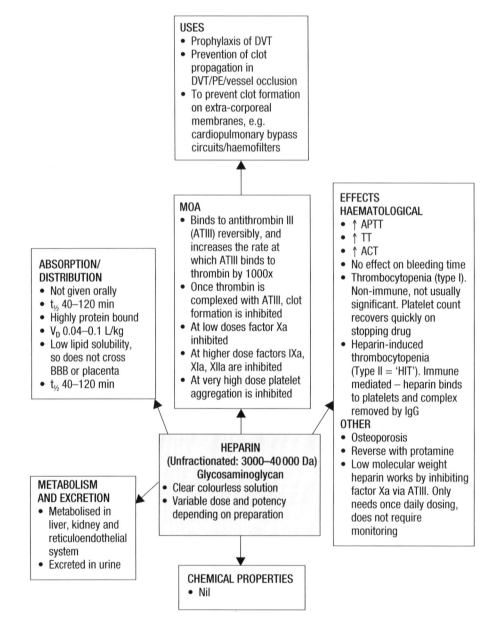

USES
- Prophylaxis of DVT
- Prevention of clot propagation in DVT/PE/vessel occlusion
- To prevent clot formation on extra-corporeal membranes, e.g. cardiopulmonary bypass circuits/haemofilters

MOA
- Binds to antithrombin III (ATIII) reversibly, and increases the rate at which ATIII binds to thrombin by 1000x
- Once thrombin is complexed with ATIII, clot formation is inhibited
- At low doses factor Xa inhibited
- At higher dose factors IXa, XIa, XIIa are inhibited
- At very high dose platelet aggregation is inhibited

ABSORPTION/ DISTRIBUTION
- Not given orally
- $t_{1/2}$ 40–120 min
- Highly protein bound
- V_D 0.04–0.1 L/kg
- Low lipid solubility, so does not cross BBB or placenta
- $t_{1/2}$ 40–120 min

EFFECTS HAEMATOLOGICAL
- ↑ APTT
- ↑ TT
- ↑ ACT
- No effect on bleeding time
- Thrombocytopenia (type I). Non-immune, not usually significant. Platelet count recovers quickly on stopping drug
- Heparin-induced thrombocytopenia (Type II = 'HIT'). Immune mediated – heparin binds to platelets and complex removed by IgG

OTHER
- Osteoporosis
- Reverse with protamine
- Low molecular weight heparin works by inhibiting factor Xa via ATIII. Only needs once daily dosing, does not require monitoring

HEPARIN (Unfractionated: 3000–40 000 Da) Glycosaminoglycan
- Clear colourless solution
- Variable dose and potency depending on preparation

METABOLISM AND EXCRETION
- Metabolised in liver, kidney and reticuloendothelial system
- Excreted in urine

CHEMICAL PROPERTIES
- Nil

WARFARIN

USES
- Prophylaxis of DVT/PE
- Prophylaxis of clot formation on prosthetic heart valves/in AF
- Prevention of clot propagation in DVT/PE/vessel occlusion

MOA
- Inhibits synthesis of vitamin K dependent clotting factors: II, VII, IX, X

Reduced Vit K   Oxidised Vit K

NAD+   NADH

Warfarin stops this

- Precursors of clotting factors synthesised in liver. They are then carboxylated and during this reaction Vit K is oxidised
- Warfarin prevents Vit K returning to its reduced state
- Only affects synthesis of new factors, takes 72 hours to work
- Action irreversible

ABSORPTION/ DISTRIBUTION
- Well absorbed orally
- Protein binding 99%
- V_D 0.1–0.16 L/kg
- $t_{1/2}$ 35–45 hours

EFFECTS HAEMATOLOGICAL
- ↑ PT
- ↑ INR

DRUG INTERACTIONS
- Availability affected by drugs which induce/inhibit liver enzymes
- Cholestyramine decreases absorption of fat soluble vitamins A, D E, and K therefore potentiates effect of warfarin

OTHER
- Hypersensitivity reactions
- Teratogenic in first trimester
- Crosses placenta and can cause fetal haemorrhage

PRE-OP
- Stop warfarin 1 week before elective surgery– replace with heparin if necessary. INR should be < 2 to operate
- Rapid reversal: beryplex/FFP
- Slow reversal (12 hours): Vit K

METABOLISM AND EXCRETION
- Hepatic metabolism
- Excreted in urine and faeces

WARFARIN Coumarin derivative
- Tablets: 0.5/1/3/5 mg

DOSE
- Patient-specific, titrate to effect
- Usually 2–9 mg/day

CHEMICAL PROPERTIES
- Nil

CHAPTER 30

Anticonvulsants

What is epilepsy and how is it classified?

Epilepsy is a chronic disease resulting from paroxysmal, episodic, abnormal and spontaneous discharge of electrical activity in the brain. It can be classified as follows:

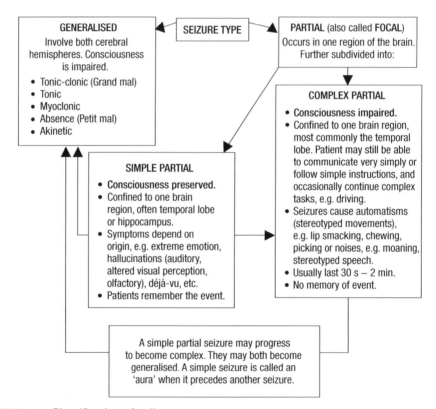

FIGURE 1.40 Classification of epilepsy

Which drugs are available to treat epilepsy and how do they work?

There are a wide variety of anticonvulsants available, but their mechanisms of action can be divided into two main groups:

➤ **Drugs enhancing GABA-mediated inhibition:**
  - benzodiazepines
  - barbiturates
  - sodium valproate
  - vigabatrin.

➤ **Drugs modulating sodium flux in nerves:**
  - phenytoin
  - carbamazepine.

This latter group of drugs exert their effect by binding to inactivated fast Na^+ channels, reducing the flux of Na^+ into cells and stabilising their membranes. Ca^{2+} and K^+ efflux is also reduced. Their anticonvulsant effect is probably achieved by preventing the repetitive opening and closing of fast Na^+ channels, so that the sodium current is reduced until it no longer provokes an action potential.

Benzodiazepines, e.g. diazepam
Benzodiazepines (BDZ) appear to have their own specific receptors, which are closely coupled to the $GABA_A$ receptor. When a BDZ binds it facilitates the binding of GABA to its respective receptor. BDZs exert their effect by increasing the frequency of opening of the $GABA_A$ channels. There are two types of BDZ receptor:
➤ **BDZ1** found in the spinal cord and cerebellum. Stimulation causes anxiolysis.
➤ **BDZ2** found in the spinal cord, hippocampus and cerebral cortex. Stimulation causes sedation and has an anticonvulsant effect.

Barbiturates, e.g. phenobarbitone
Barbiturates increase the duration of opening of the $GABA_A$ chloride channel when stimulated.

Vigabatrin: This reversibly inhibits GABA transaminase, the enzyme which breaks down GABA.

How would you anaesthetise a patient with epilespsy?
Pre-operative assessment: Take a full and through anaesthetic history, paying close attention to the following:
➤ History of the epileptic activity.
➤ Underlying pathology or lesion causing the seizures.
➤ Type, frequency and duration of the seizures and when the last one occurred.
➤ Occupation and driving status.
➤ Drug history. It is important that the patient receives their medication in a timely manner. If they are nil by mouth for any prolonged period, appropriate medication should be given by an alternative route, e.g. rectally or intravenously. This should be discussed with a neurologist.

Perioperative care:
➤ Induce anaesthesia using thiopentone.
➤ Avoid ketamine and etomidate as they can lower the seizure threshold.
➤ Anticonvulsants induce liver enzyme activity and therefore the patient may need increased doses of anaesthetic agents and muscle relaxants.
➤ Avoid hypoxia and hypercapnia throughout the procedure as these states can lower the seizure threshold.

Propofol is said to cause epileptiform movements, but it has not been shown to produce epileptiform activity on the EEG. In some units it is used in the treatment of status epilepticus and so it is probably safe for routine use in patients with epilepsy.

Describe the GABA receptor
GABA (gamma amino-butyric acid) is the main inhibitory neurotransmitter in the CNS. The activation of the GABA receptor causes increased flux of chloride or potassium ions into the

cell and causes hyperpolarisation of the membrane, therefore stabilising the synapse. There are 2 GABA receptor subtypes:

➤ **GABA$_A$:** A ligand-gated chloride ion channel, with five receptor subunits (2α, β, δ and γ) arranged around the ion channel. These are found on the post-synaptic membrane.

➤ **GABA$_B$:** A G-protein coupled receptor. Stimulation of GABA$_B$ causes increased potassium conductance. These are found on both the pre– and postsynaptic membranes. Baclofen acts via these receptors.

PHENYTOIN

USES
- Treatment and prophylaxis of tonic-clonic seizures
- Trigeminal neuralgia
- Antiarrhythmic (Class 1b) used to treat ventricular arrhythmias of tricyclic and digoxin overdose

MOA
- Binds to inactivated fast Na^+ channels reducing flux of Na^+ into cells and stabilising the membrane
- Ca^{2+} and K^+ efflux also reduced
- Anticonvulsant effect probably achieved by preventing repetitive opening and closing of fast Na channels, so that the sodium current is reduced until it no longer provokes an action potential

EFFECTS
CVS
- Class 1b shortens refractory period of cardiac muscle. Rapid injection can cause heart block, VF and asystole

CNS
- Antiepileptic

SIDE-EFFECTS
Idiosyncratic:
- Hirsuitism
- Coarse facies
- Acne
- Gum hyperplasia
- Megaloblastic anaemia
- Aplastic anaemia
- Rashes
- SLE
- Peripheral neuropathy

Concentration-dependent:
- Nausea and vomiting
- Tremor
- Ataxia
- Nystagmus
- Vertigo
- Drowsiness

Teratogenicity:
- Craniofacial abnormalities
- Limb abnormalities
- Cardiac abnormalities
- Growth retardation

ABSORPTION/ DISTRIBUTION
- Oral bioavailability 90%
- Protein binding 90%
- V_D 0.5 L/kg

METABOLISM AND EXCRETION
- Hepatic metabolism
- Exhibits **zero order kinetics** just above therapeutic range so care should be taken with dosing so as not to cause toxicity
- 80% renally excreted
- Potent liver enzyme inducer, so check for drug interactions
- Increases the required dose of aminosteroid muscle relaxants by 80%
- May decrease MAC of volatiles

PHENYTOIN
Anticonvulsant
Class 1b antiarrhythmic
- Capsules: 25/50/100/300 mg
- Syrup: 6 mg/mL
- Solution: 50 mg/mL

DOSE
- Loading: 15 mg/kg for treatment of seizure
- Maintenance: 100 mg 8 hourly
- Oral dose: 200–600 mg daily
- Therapeutic range: 10–20 mg/L

CHEMICAL PROPERTIES
- Nil

SODIUM VALPROATE

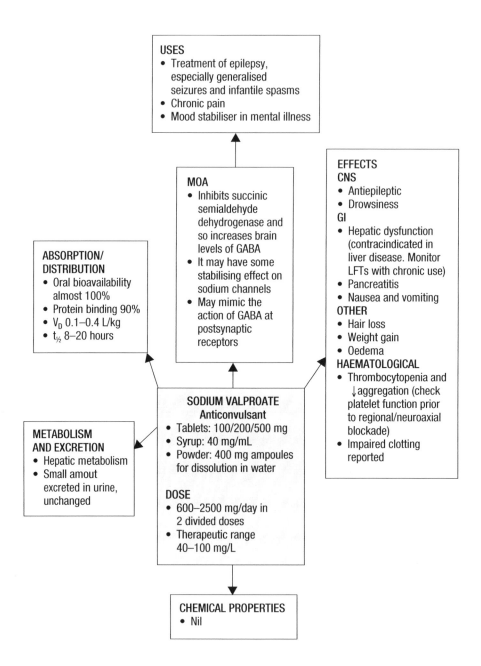

USES
- Treatment of epilepsy, especially generalised seizures and infantile spasms
- Chronic pain
- Mood stabiliser in mental illness

MOA
- Inhibits succinic semialdehyde dehydrogenase and so increases brain levels of GABA
- It may have some stabilising effect on sodium channels
- May mimic the action of GABA at postsynaptic receptors

EFFECTS
CNS
- Antiepileptic
- Drowsiness
GI
- Hepatic dysfunction (contracindicated in liver disease. Monitor LFTs with chronic use)
- Pancreatitis
- Nausea and vomiting
OTHER
- Hair loss
- Weight gain
- Oedema
HAEMATOLOGICAL
- Thrombocytopenia and ↓aggregation (check platelet function prior to regional/neuroaxial blockade)
- Impaired clotting reported

ABSORPTION/ DISTRIBUTION
- Oral bioavailability almost 100%
- Protein binding 90%
- V_D 0.1–0.4 L/kg
- $t_{1/2}$ 8–20 hours

METABOLISM AND EXCRETION
- Hepatic metabolism
- Small amout excreted in urine, unchanged

SODIUM VALPROATE
Anticonvulsant
- Tablets: 100/200/500 mg
- Syrup: 40 mg/mL
- Powder: 400 mg ampoules for dissolution in water

DOSE
- 600–2500 mg/day in 2 divided doses
- Therapeutic range 40–100 mg/L

CHEMICAL PROPERTIES
- Nil

CARBAMAZEPINE

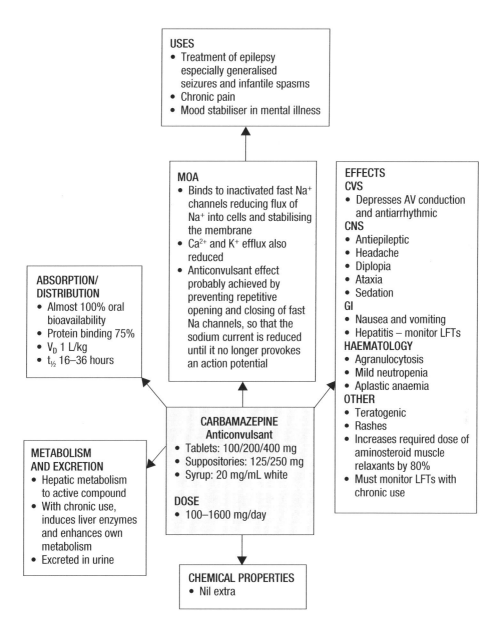

USES
- Treatment of epilepsy especially generalised seizures and infantile spasms
- Chronic pain
- Mood stabiliser in mental illness

MOA
- Binds to inactivated fast Na^+ channels reducing flux of Na^+ into cells and stabilising the membrane
- Ca^{2+} and K^+ efflux also reduced
- Anticonvulsant effect probably achieved by preventing repetitive opening and closing of fast Na channels, so that the sodium current is reduced until it no longer provokes an action potential

EFFECTS
CVS
- Depresses AV conduction and antiarrhythmic
CNS
- Antiepileptic
- Headache
- Diplopia
- Ataxia
- Sedation
GI
- Nausea and vomiting
- Hepatitis – monitor LFTs
HAEMATOLOGY
- Agranulocytosis
- Mild neutropenia
- Aplastic anaemia
OTHER
- Teratogenic
- Rashes
- Increases required dose of aminosteroid muscle relaxants by 80%
- Must monitor LFTs with chronic use

ABSORPTION/ DISTRIBUTION
- Almost 100% oral bioavailability
- Protein binding 75%
- V_D 1 L/kg
- $t_{1/2}$ 16–36 hours

METABOLISM AND EXCRETION
- Hepatic metabolism to active compound
- With chronic use, induces liver enzymes and enhances own metabolism
- Excreted in urine

CARBAMAZEPINE
Anticonvulsant
- Tablets: 100/200/400 mg
- Suppositories: 125/250 mg
- Syrup: 20 mg/mL white

DOSE
- 100–1600 mg/day

CHEMICAL PROPERTIES
- Nil extra

CHAPTER 31

Drugs used to treat asthma

Asthma is a common disease characterised by reversible airway obstruction secondary to bronchoconstriction. It is a potentially life-threatening condition causing approximately 1500 deaths per year in the UK.

Anaesthetists will regularly anaesthetise patients with asthma and also be involved in the management of the patient with severe or life-threatening asthma. Thus a thorough understanding of the pathophysiology of asthma and its treatment is expected.

Describe the pathophysiology of severe and life-threatening asthma

➤ Bronchospasm from a combination of bronchial smooth muscle constriction, inflammation and mucus production.

➤ Common triggers include allergens (e.g. house dust mite), tobacco smoke, cold air, exercise, viral infection and, in some patients, drugs such as non-steroidal anti-inflammatory drugs or β blockers.

➤ Bronchoconstriction is mediated by the parasympathetic nervous system – acetylcholine released from vagal afferent nerve endings leads to a rise in cyclic GMP and hence intracellular calcium levels, causing bronchial smooth muscle contraction.

➤ Bronchoconstriction results in increased airways resistance and reduced expiratory gas flow, leading to dynamic hyperinflation of the lungs and the generation of intrinsic positive airway pressure.

➤ Type 1 respiratory failure ensues in the early stages of an acute episode primarily due to ventilation-perfusion mismatching. However, type 2 respiratory failure may develop as the patient becomes exhausted from the increased work of breathing, an ominous sign.

Outline the pharmacological management of asthma

The aim of pharmacological management of asthma is disease control as defined by absence of symptoms, no limitations on activities and normal lung function. A step-wise approach is adopted, with therapy titrated to severity:

➤ **Step 1:** Mild intermittent asthma – inhaled short-acting B_2 agonist (e.g. salbutamol) as required.

➤ **Step 2:** Regular preventative therapy – add inhaled steroid 200–800 mcg/day.

➤ **Step 3:** Initial add-on therapy – add inhaled long-acting B_2 agonist (e.g. salmeterol). Assess response and if good then continue. If improvement seen but control still inadequate, increase inhaled steroid dose; but if no improvement seen, discontinue long acting B_2 agonist and increase inhaled steroid and consider other therapies such as leukotriene receptor antagonist (e.g. montelukast) or slow-release theophylline.

Leukotriene receptor antagonists block the bronchoconstricting effects of leukotrienes on the airways and act synergistically with inhaled steroids. This class of drug is especially of benefit in exercise-induced asthma. Churg–Strauss syndrome (eosinophilia, vasculitic rash, pulmonary infiltrates) is a rare association with the use of leukotriene receptor antagonists.

➤ **Step 4:** Persistent poor control – consider trial of increasing inhaled steroid, addition of a fourth drug, e.g. leukotriene receptor antagonist, slow release theophylline or β_2 agonist tablet.

➤ **Step 5:** Continuous or frequent use of oral steroid – refer to specialist care.

Discuss the drug treatment of severe and life-threatening asthma

Treatment of severe and life-threatening asthma involves correcting the hypoxaemia and reduction of airways resistance through bronchodilation.

1 **Oxygen** – initially commence high concentration oxygen and then titrate to maintain $S_aO_2 > 92\%$. Hypoxia is the commonest cause of death in life-threatening asthma.

2 **β_2 receptor agonists (nebulised)** – oxygen driven nebulisation of salbutamol 2.5–5.0 mg back to back initially. Drug delivered to the bronchioles is only a small percentage of the total administered dose, due to bronchoconstriction.

3 **Muscarinic antagonist (nebulised)** – oxygen driven nebulisation of ipratropium bromide 500 µg 6 hourly.

4 **Steroids** – depending on the clinical situation administer either 40 mg of prednisolone orally or 200 mg of hydrocortisone intravenously followed by 50–100 mg of hydrocortisone 6 hourly.

5 **Magnesium sulphate** – administer 2 g over 20 min intravenously. Side-effects include hypotension and muscle weakness, however being an excellent smooth muscle dilator it has an important role in the management of asthma.

6 **Intravenous β_2 agonist** – salbutamol may be administered as an infusion at a rate of 5–20 µg/min, but this is not without potential serious systemic effects such as severe tachycardia and lactic acidosis.

7 **Intravenous phosphodiesterase inhibitor** – aminophylline loading dose of 5 mg/kg followed by an infusion at 0.5 mg/kg/min. Omit the loading dose in those patients already taking oral theophylline (narrow therapeutic index). Aminophylline acts by blocking the enzyme phosphodiesterase thereby increasing intracellular levels of cyclic AMP, which reduces intracellular calcium within the bronchial smooth muscle leading to bronchodilation. The role of phosphodiesterase inhibitors in the treatment of acute life-threatening asthma has recently been questioned, as there is evidence to suggest it may not be effective and may even be harmful because of the drug side-effect profile (specifically cardiac arrhythmias). Plasma aminophylline levels should be monitored during its use.

8 **Adrenaline** – an excellent bronchodilator through its β agonist action. It should be considered in resistant bronchospasm. It may be administered via nebulisation (1:1000 adrenaline) or in extremis via the intravenous route (titrated 100 mcg intravenous boluses).

9 **Heliox** – a mixture of helium and oxygen (commonly 30% oxygen/70% helium). The low density of this gas mixture improves gas flow within the airways by converting turbulent flow to laminar flow, thereby reducing work of breathing. It may be used in non-life-threatening asthma but its use is limited by the fractional inspired oxygen concentration.

10 **Ketamine** – an NMDA receptor antagonist with excellent bronchodilating properties. It may be used to induce anaesthesia in patients with life-threatening asthma and may be used for sedation and treatment of bronchoconstriction in ventilated patients.

11 **Inhalational volatile anaesthetics** – sevoflurane is a good bronchodilator and may be used in resistant bronchospasm. Delivery usually requires an anaesthetic machine although it may be administered through in-line devices in certain critical care

ventilators. Gas analysis and scavenging are essential requirements when using volatile agents.

Which drugs should be avoided in acute severe/life-threatening asthma?
- β-blockers.
- NSAIDs.
- Caution with thiopentone which may cause histamine release.
- Avoid atracurium which causes histamine release.
- Caution with morphine which causes histamine release.

SALBUTAMOL

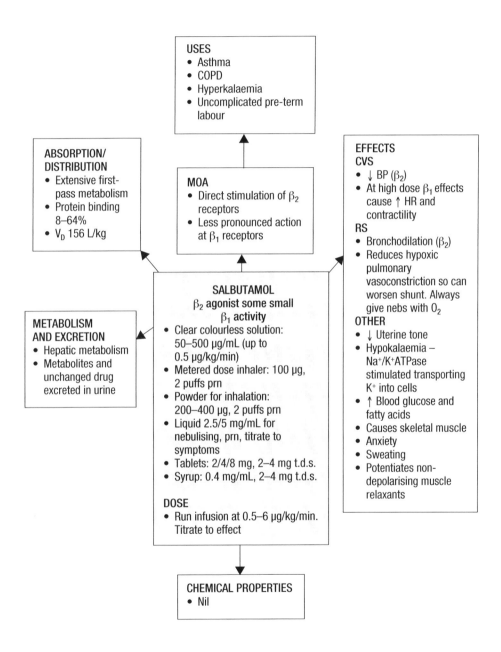

USES
- Asthma
- COPD
- Hyperkalaemia
- Uncomplicated pre-term labour

ABSORPTION/ DISTRIBUTION
- Extensive first-pass metabolism
- Protein binding 8–64%
- V_D 156 L/kg

MOA
- Direct stimulation of β_2 receptors
- Less pronounced action at β_1 receptors

EFFECTS
CVS
- $\downarrow$ BP (β_2)
- At high dose β_1 effects cause $\uparrow$ HR and contractility

RS
- Bronchodilation (β_2)
- Reduces hypoxic pulmonary vasoconstriction so can worsen shunt. Always give nebs with O_2

OTHER
- $\downarrow$ Uterine tone
- Hypokalaemia – Na^+/K^+ATPase stimulated transporting K^+ into cells
- $\uparrow$ Blood glucose and fatty acids
- Causes skeletal muscle
- Anxiety
- Sweating
- Potentiates non-depolarising muscle relaxants

METABOLISM AND EXCRETION
- Hepatic metabolism
- Metabolites and unchanged drug excreted in urine

SALBUTAMOL
β_2 **agonist some small** β_1 **activity**
- Clear colourless solution: 50–500 µg/mL (up to 0.5 µg/kg/min)
- Metered dose inhaler: 100 µg, 2 puffs prn
- Powder for inhalation: 200–400 µg, 2 puffs prn
- Liquid 2.5/5 mg/mL for nebulising, prn, titrate to symptoms
- Tablets: 2/4/8 mg, 2–4 mg t.d.s.
- Syrup: 0.4 mg/mL, 2–4 mg t.d.s.

DOSE
- Run infusion at 0.5–6 µg/kg/min. Titrate to effect

CHEMICAL PROPERTIES
- Nil

AMINOPHYLLINE

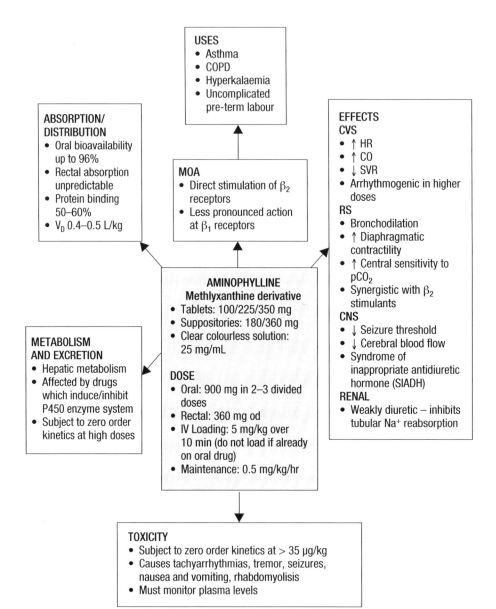

USES
- Asthma
- COPD
- Hyperkalaemia
- Uncomplicated pre-term labour

ABSORPTION/ DISTRIBUTION
- Oral bioavailability up to 96%
- Rectal absorption unpredictable
- Protein binding 50–60%
- V_D 0.4–0.5 L/kg

MOA
- Direct stimulation of β_2 receptors
- Less pronounced action at β_1 receptors

EFFECTS

CVS
- ↑ HR
- ↑ CO
- ↓ SVR
- Arrhythmogenic in higher doses

RS
- Bronchodilation
- ↑ Diaphragmatic contractility
- ↑ Central sensitivity to pCO_2
- Synergistic with β_2 stimulants

CNS
- ↓ Seizure threshold
- ↓ Cerebral blood flow
- Syndrome of inappropriate antidiuretic hormone (SIADH)

RENAL
- Weakly diuretic – inhibits tubular Na^+ reabsorption

AMINOPHYLLINE
Methlyxanthine derivative
- Tablets: 100/225/350 mg
- Suppositories: 180/360 mg
- Clear colourless solution: 25 mg/mL

DOSE
- Oral: 900 mg in 2–3 divided doses
- Rectal: 360 mg od
- IV Loading: 5 mg/kg over 10 min (do not load if already on oral drug)
- Maintenance: 0.5 mg/kg/hr

METABOLISM AND EXCRETION
- Hepatic metabolism
- Affected by drugs which induce/inhibit P450 enzyme system
- Subject to zero order kinetics at high doses

TOXICITY
- Subject to zero order kinetics at > 35 µg/kg
- Causes tachyarrhythmias, tremor, seizures, nausea and vomiting, rhabdomyolisis
- Must monitor plasma levels

CHAPTER 32

Miscellaneous drugs

Benzodiazepines

DIAZEPAM

USES
- Tonic-clonic seizures and status epilepticus
- Anxiolysis
- Alcohol withdrawal
- Muscle spasm
- Sedation
- Premed

ABSORPTION/ DISTRIBUTION
- Oral bioavailability up to 100% as very lipid soluble
- Protein binding 99%
- V_D 0.8–1.4 L/kg
- Active metabolites have $t_{1/2}$ >100 hours!

MOA
- Agonist at the benzodiazepine receptor which is coupled to GABA receptor
- Stimulation causes ↑ frequency of opening of GABA's Cl- ion channel
- This causes hyperpolarisation and stabilisation of membrane by increasing flux of Cl- ions into cell

EFFECTS
CVS
- Slight, transient ↓ BP
- ↑ Coronary artery vasodilation
- ↓ Myocardial oxygen demand

RS
- ↓ RR
- Apnoea in high doses

CNS
- Anticonvulsant
- Hypnosis
- Sedation
- Anxiolysis
- Amnesia (anterograde)
- ↓ MAC
- Drowsiness
- Ataxia
- Tolerance and dependence

METABOLISM AND EXCRETION
- Hepatic metabolism to active compounds
  - Desmethyldiazepam,
  - Oxazepam and
  - Temazepam
- Metabolites excreted in urine

DIAZEPAM
Benzodiazepine
- Tablets: 2/5/10 mg
- IV white solution: 2/4 mg/mL

DOSE
- IV for sedation: 5–20 mg, titrate to effect
- Alcohol withdrawal: 20–30 mg q.d.s., reducing dose regime
- Status epilepticus: 10 mg IV or PR repeated prn

CHEMICAL PROPERTIES
- Nil

MIDAZOLAM

USES
- Sedation
- Anxiolysis
- With morphine for induction of anaesthesia in unstable patients

ABSORPTION/ DISTRIBUTION
- Oral bioavailability ~ 40%
- Protein binding 95%
- High hepatic extraction ratio, so if hepatic blood flow is poor/poor liver function, half-life will increase
- $t_{1/2}$ 1–4 hours
- Shorter action than other BDZs because of redistribution

MOA
- Benzodiazepine receptor coupled to GABA receptor
- Stimulation causes ↑ frequency of opening of GABA's Cl⁻ ion channel
- Causes hyperpolarisation of membrane by increasing flux of Cl⁻ ions into cell

EFFECTS
CVS
- ↓ SVR by one-third
- ↑ HR
- Obtunds response to laryngoscopy when combined with opioid

RS
- ↑ RR
- ↓ V_T
- No change in MV
- Apnoea in some
- Blunts response to pCO_2

CNS
- Hypnosis
- Sedation
- Anxiolysis
- Amnesia (anterograde)
- ↓ Cerebral metabolic oxygen requirements
- ↓ Cerebral blood flow
- ↓ MAC by 15%

GI
- ↓ Hepatic blood flow

GU
- ↓ Renal blood flow

METABOLISM AND EXCRETION
- Hepatic metabolism
- Hydroxylation to 1α hydroxymidazolam (active). This is conjugated and excreted in urine
- <5% converted to oxazepam
- Alfentanil metabolised by same enzymes (P4503A3/4) therefore they may potentiate each other's effects

MIDAZOLAM
Imidazolbenzodiazepine
- Clear colourless solution: 1/2/5 mg/mL
- Oral/nasal/PR/IM/IV/ intrathecally/epidural

DOSE
- Oral: 0.5 mg/kg (max 20 mg)
- IV: 0.02–0.1 mg/kg for sedation, titrate to effect
- Spinal: 0.3–2 mg
- Epidural: 0.1–0.2 mg/kg

CHEMICAL PROPERTIES
- Contains tautomeric diazepine ring structure
- The ring can be open or closed depending on ambient pH
  - > 4 ring closed = non-ionised and lipid soluble
  - < 4 ring open = ionised and less lipid soluble
- pH in ampoule = 3
- pKa = 8.5 so at pH 7.4, 89% un-ionised
- Drug is water soluble, so no pain on injection
- Effects can be reversed with flumazenil

TEMAZEPAM

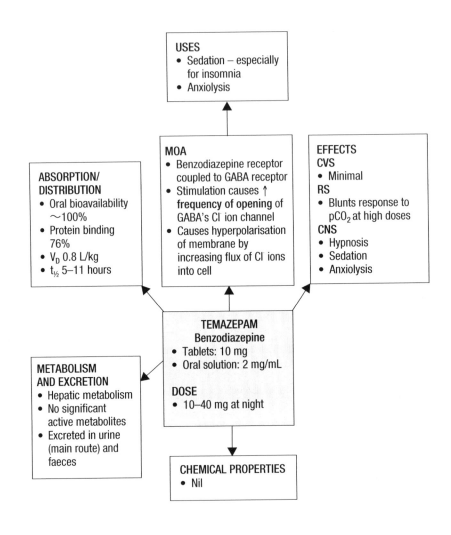

USES
- Sedation – especially for insomnia
- Anxiolysis

MOA
- Benzodiazepine receptor coupled to GABA receptor
- Stimulation causes ↑ **frequency of opening** of GABA's Cl ion channel
- Causes hyperpolarisation of membrane by increasing flux of Cl ions into cell

EFFECTS
CVS
- Minimal
RS
- Blunts response to pCO_2 at high doses
CNS
- Hypnosis
- Sedation
- Anxiolysis

ABSORPTION/ DISTRIBUTION
- Oral bioavailability ~100%
- Protein binding 76%
- V_D 0.8 L/kg
- $t_{1/2}$ 5–11 hours

TEMAZEPAM
Benzodiazepine
- Tablets: 10 mg
- Oral solution: 2 mg/mL

DOSE
- 10–40 mg at night

METABOLISM AND EXCRETION
- Hepatic metabolism
- No significant active metabolites
- Excreted in urine (main route) and faeces

CHEMICAL PROPERTIES
- Nil

FLUMAZENIL

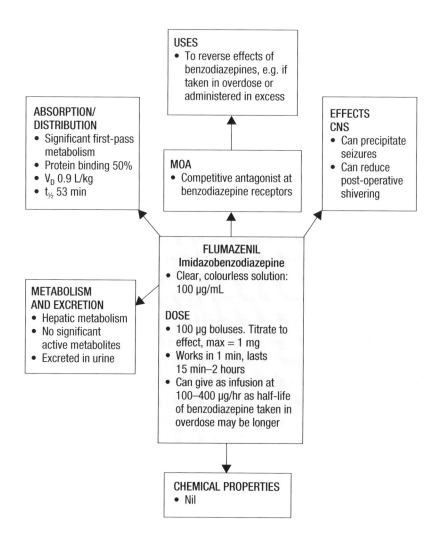

USES
- To reverse effects of benzodiazepines, e.g. if taken in overdose or administered in excess

ABSORPTION/ DISTRIBUTION
- Significant first-pass metabolism
- Protein binding 50%
- V_D 0.9 L/kg
- $t_{1/2}$ 53 min

MOA
- Competitive antagonist at benzodiazepine receptors

EFFECTS CNS
- Can precipitate seizures
- Can reduce post-operative shivering

FLUMAZENIL
Imidazobenzodiazepine
- Clear, colourless solution: 100 μg/mL

DOSE
- 100 μg boluses. Titrate to effect, max = 1 mg
- Works in 1 min, lasts 15 min–2 hours
- Can give as infusion at 100–400 μg/hr as half-life of benzodiazepine taken in overdose may be longer

METABOLISM AND EXCRETION
- Hepatic metabolism
- No significant active metabolites
- Excreted in urine

CHEMICAL PROPERTIES
- Nil

Vasopressors and inotropes

PHENYLEPHRINE

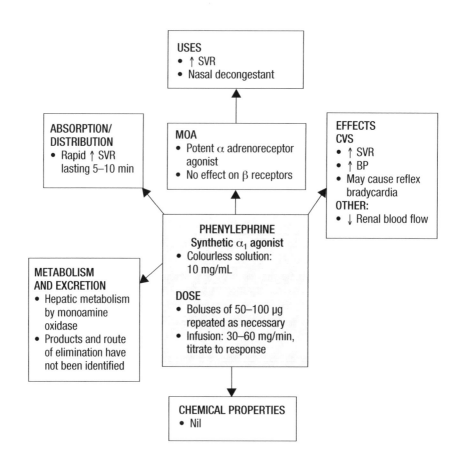

USES
- ↑ SVR
- Nasal decongestant

ABSORPTION/
DISTRIBUTION
- Rapid ↑ SVR
  lasting 5–10 min

MOA
- Potent α adrenoreceptor agonist
- No effect on β receptors

EFFECTS
CVS
- ↑ SVR
- ↑ BP
- May cause reflex bradycardia
OTHER:
- ↓ Renal blood flow

PHENYLEPHRINE
Synthetic α_1 agonist
- Colourless solution: 10 mg/mL

DOSE
- Boluses of 50–100 μg repeated as necessary
- Infusion: 30–60 mg/min, titrate to response

METABOLISM
AND EXCRETION
- Hepatic metabolism by monoamine oxidase
- Products and route of elimination have not been identified

CHEMICAL PROPERTIES
- Nil

METARAMINOL

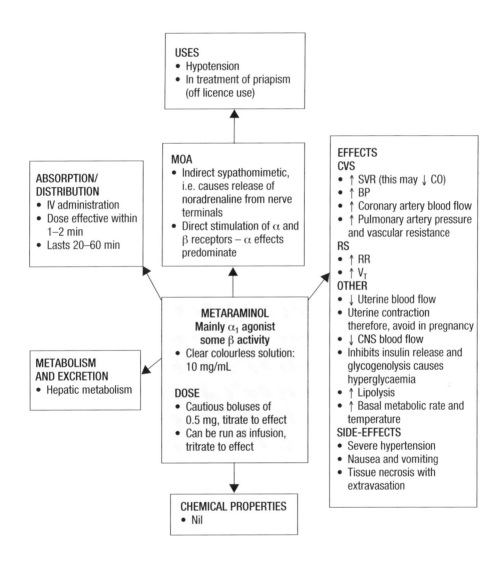

USES
- Hypotension
- In treatment of priapism (off licence use)

ABSORPTION/ DISTRIBUTION
- IV administration
- Dose effective within 1–2 min
- Lasts 20–60 min

MOA
- Indirect sypathomimetic, i.e. causes release of noradrenaline from nerve terminals
- Direct stimulation of α and β receptors – α effects predominate

METABOLISM AND EXCRETION
- Hepatic metabolism

METARAMINOL
Mainly α_1 agonist
some β activity
- Clear colourless solution: 10 mg/mL

DOSE
- Cautious boluses of 0.5 mg, titrate to effect
- Can be run as infusion, tritrate to effect

EFFECTS
CVS
- ↑ SVR (this may ↓ CO)
- ↑ BP
- ↑ Coronary artery blood flow
- ↑ Pulmonary artery pressure and vascular resistance

RS
- ↑ RR
- ↑ V_T

OTHER
- ↓ Uterine blood flow
- Uterine contraction therefore, avoid in pregnancy
- ↓ CNS blood flow
- Inhibits insulin release and glycogenolysis causes hyperglycaemia
- ↑ Lipolysis
- ↑ Basal metabolic rate and temperature

SIDE-EFFECTS
- Severe hypertension
- Nausea and vomiting
- Tissue necrosis with extravasation

CHEMICAL PROPERTIES
- Nil

NORADRENALINE

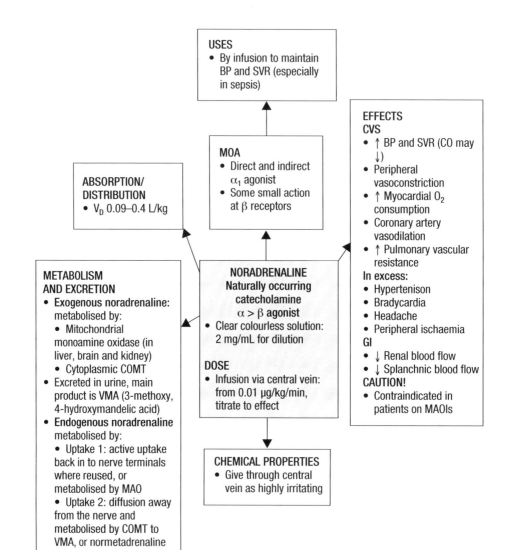

USES
- By infusion to maintain BP and SVR (especially in sepsis)

MOA
- Direct and indirect α_1 agonist
- Some small action at β receptors

ABSORPTION/ DISTRIBUTION
- V_D 0.09–0.4 L/kg

METABOLISM AND EXCRETION
- Exogenous noradrenaline: metabolised by:
  - Mitochondrial monoamine oxidase (in liver, brain and kidney)
  - Cytoplasmic COMT
- Excreted in urine, main product is VMA (3-methoxy, 4-hydroxymandelic acid)
- Endogenous noradrenaline metabolised by:
  - Uptake 1: active uptake back in to nerve terminals where reused, or metabolised by MAO
  - Uptake 2: diffusion away from the nerve and metabolised by COMT to VMA, or normetadrenaline

NORADRENALINE
Naturally occurring catecholamine
$\alpha > \beta$ agonist
- Clear colourless solution: 2 mg/mL for dilution

DOSE
- Infusion via central vein: from 0.01 µg/kg/min, titrate to effect

EFFECTS
CVS
- ↑ BP and SVR (CO may ↓)
- Peripheral vasoconstriction
- ↑ Myocardial O_2 consumption
- Coronary artery vasodilation
- ↑ Pulmonary vascular resistance

In excess:
- Hypertenison
- Bradycardia
- Headache
- Peripheral ischaemia

GI
- ↓ Renal blood flow
- ↓ Splanchnic blood flow

CAUTION!
- Contraindicated in patients on MAOIs

CHEMICAL PROPERTIES
- Give through central vein as highly irritating

EPHEDRINE

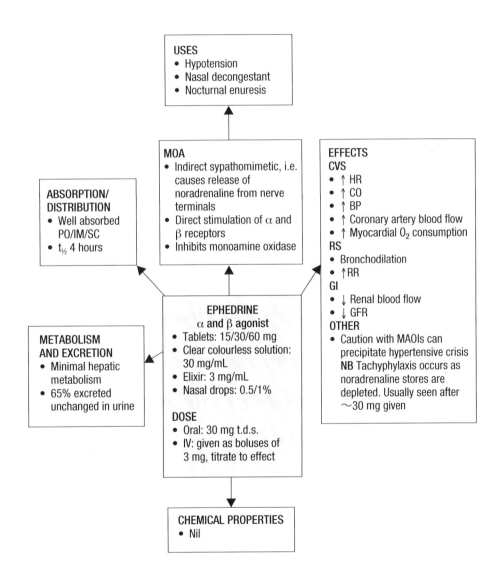

USES
- Hypotension
- Nasal decongestant
- Nocturnal enuresis

MOA
- Indirect sypathomimetic, i.e. causes release of noradrenaline from nerve terminals
- Direct stimulation of α and β receptors
- Inhibits monoamine oxidase

ABSORPTION/ DISTRIBUTION
- Well absorbed PO/IM/SC
- $t_{1/2}$ 4 hours

EFFECTS
CVS
- ↑ HR
- ↑ CO
- ↑ BP
- ↑ Coronary artery blood flow
- ↑ Myocardial O_2 consumption
RS
- Bronchodilation
- ↑RR
GI
- ↓ Renal blood flow
- ↓ GFR
OTHER
- Caution with MAOIs can precipitate hypertensive crisis
NB Tachyphylaxis occurs as noradrenaline stores are depleted. Usually seen after ~30 mg given

EPHEDRINE
α and β agonist
- Tablets: 15/30/60 mg
- Clear colourless solution: 30 mg/mL
- Elixir: 3 mg/mL
- Nasal drops: 0.5/1%

DOSE
- Oral: 30 mg t.d.s.
- IV: given as boluses of 3 mg, titrate to effect

METABOLISM AND EXCRETION
- Minimal hepatic metabolism
- 65% excreted unchanged in urine

CHEMICAL PROPERTIES
- Nil

ADRENALINE

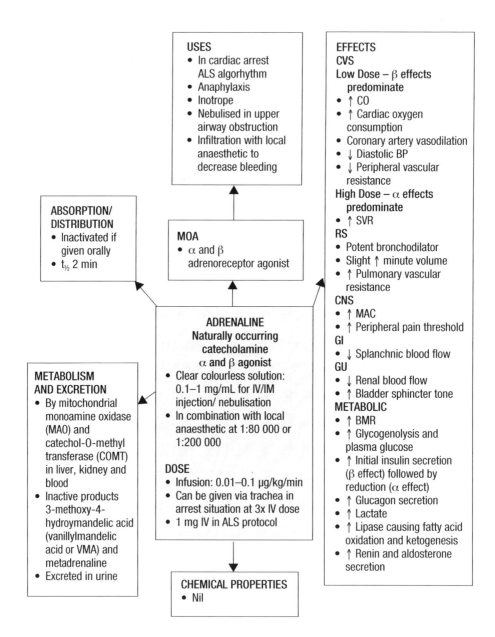

USES
- In cardiac arrest ALS algorhythm
- Anaphylaxis
- Inotrope
- Nebulised in upper airway obstruction
- Infiltration with local anaesthetic to decrease bleeding

EFFECTS
CVS
Low Dose – β effects predominate
- ↑ CO
- ↑ Cardiac oxygen consumption
- Coronary artery vasodilation
- ↓ Diastolic BP
- ↓ Peripheral vascular resistance

High Dose – α effects predominate
- ↑ SVR

RS
- Potent bronchodilator
- Slight ↑ minute volume
- ↑ Pulmonary vascular resistance

CNS
- ↑ MAC
- ↑ Peripheral pain threshold

GI
- ↓ Splanchnic blood flow

GU
- ↓ Renal blood flow
- ↑ Bladder sphincter tone

METABOLIC
- ↑ BMR
- ↑ Glycogenolysis and plasma glucose
- ↑ Initial insulin secretion (β effect) followed by reduction (α effect)
- ↑ Glucagon secretion
- ↑ Lactate
- ↑ Lipase causing fatty acid oxidation and ketogenesis
- ↑ Renin and aldosterone secretion

ABSORPTION/ DISTRIBUTION
- Inactivated if given orally
- t½ 2 min

MOA
- α and β adrenoreceptor agonist

METABOLISM AND EXCRETION
- By mitochondrial monoamine oxidase (MAO) and catechol-O-methyl transferase (COMT) in liver, kidney and blood
- Inactive products 3-methoxy-4-hydroymandelic acid (vanillylmandelic acid or VMA) and metadrenaline
- Excreted in urine

ADRENALINE
Naturally occurring catecholamine
α and β agonist
- Clear colourless solution: 0.1–1 mg/mL for IV/IM injection/ nebulisation
- In combination with local anaesthetic at 1:80 000 or 1:200 000

DOSE
- Infusion: 0.01–0.1 μg/kg/min
- Can be given via trachea in arrest situation at 3x IV dose
- 1 mg IV in ALS protocol

CHEMICAL PROPERTIES
- Nil

DOBUTAMINE

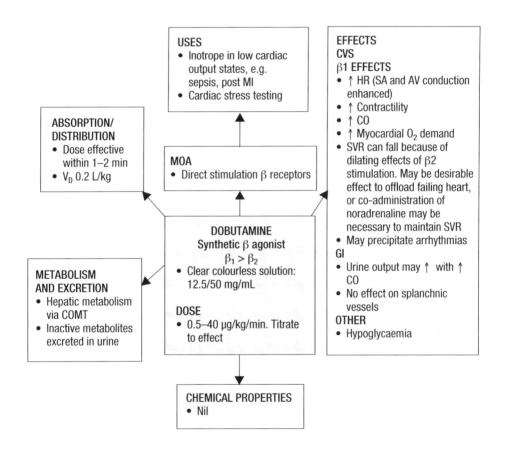

USES
- Inotrope in low cardiac output states, e.g. sepsis, post MI
- Cardiac stress testing

ABSORPTION/ DISTRIBUTION
- Dose effective within 1–2 min
- V_D 0.2 L/kg

MOA
- Direct stimulation β receptors

DOBUTAMINE
Synthetic β agonist
$\beta_1 > \beta_2$
- Clear colourless solution: 12.5/50 mg/mL

DOSE
- 0.5–40 µg/kg/min. Titrate to effect

METABOLISM AND EXCRETION
- Hepatic metabolism via COMT
- Inactive metabolites excreted in urine

EFFECTS
CVS
β1 EFFECTS
- ↑ HR (SA and AV conduction enhanced)
- ↑ Contractility
- ↑ CO
- ↑ Myocardial O_2 demand
- SVR can fall because of dilating effects of β2 stimulation. May be desirable effect to offload failing heart, or co-administration of noradrenaline may be necessary to maintain SVR
- May precipitate arrhythmias
GI
- Urine output may ↑ with ↑ CO
- No effect on splanchnic vessels
OTHER
- Hypoglycaemia

CHEMICAL PROPERTIES
- Nil

DOPAMINE

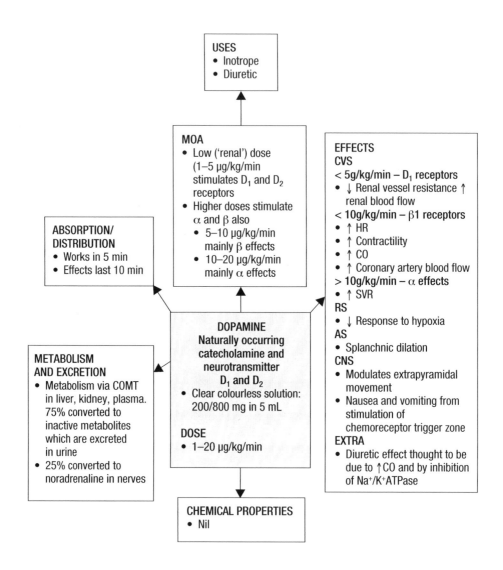

USES
- Inotrope
- Diuretic

MOA
- Low ('renal') dose (1–5 µg/kg/min stimulates D_1 and D_2 receptors
- Higher doses stimulate α and β also
  - 5–10 µg/kg/min mainly β effects
  - 10–20 µg/kg/min mainly α effects

ABSORPTION/ DISTRIBUTION
- Works in 5 min
- Effects last 10 min

DOPAMINE
Naturally occurring catecholamine and neurotransmitter
D_1 and D_2
- Clear colourless solution: 200/800 mg in 5 mL

DOSE
- 1–20 µg/kg/min

EFFECTS
CVS
< 5g/kg/min – D_1 receptors
- ↓ Renal vessel resistance ↑ renal blood flow
< 10g/kg/min – $\beta1$ receptors
- ↑ HR
- ↑ Contractility
- ↑ CO
- ↑ Coronary artery blood flow
> 10g/kg/min – α effects
- ↑ SVR
RS
- ↓ Response to hypoxia
AS
- Splanchnic dilation
CNS
- Modulates extrapyramidal movement
- Nausea and vomiting from stimulation of chemoreceptor trigger zone
EXTRA
- Diuretic effect thought to be due to ↑CO and by inhibition of Na^+/K^+ATPase

METABOLISM AND EXCRETION
- Metabolism via COMT in liver, kidney, plasma. 75% converted to inactive metabolites which are excreted in urine
- 25% converted to noradrenaline in nerves

CHEMICAL PROPERTIES
- Nil

DOPEXAMINE

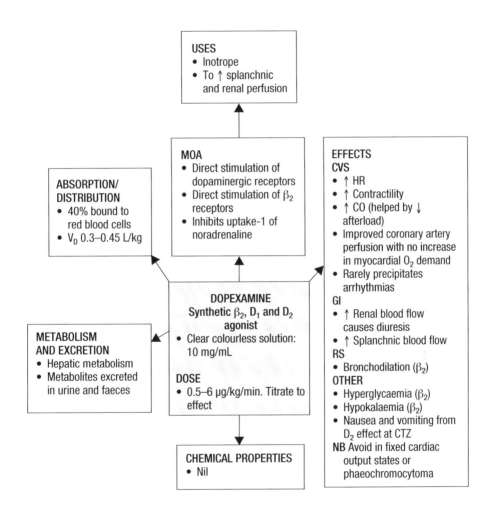

USES
- Inotrope
- To ↑ splanchnic and renal perfusion

MOA
- Direct stimulation of dopaminergic receptors
- Direct stimulation of β_2 receptors
- Inhibits uptake-1 of noradrenaline

ABSORPTION/ DISTRIBUTION
- 40% bound to red blood cells
- V_D 0.3–0.45 L/kg

EFFECTS
CVS
- ↑ HR
- ↑ Contractility
- ↑ CO (helped by ↓ afterload)
- Improved coronary artery perfusion with no increase in myocardial O_2 demand
- Rarely precipitates arrhythmias

GI
- ↑ Renal blood flow causes diuresis
- ↑ Splanchnic blood flow

RS
- Bronchodilation (β_2)

OTHER
- Hyperglycaemia (β_2)
- Hypokalaemia (β_2)
- Nausea and vomiting from D_2 effect at CTZ

NB Avoid in fixed cardiac output states or phaeochromocytoma

DOPEXAMINE
Synthetic β_2, D_1 and D_2 agonist
- Clear colourless solution: 10 mg/mL

DOSE
- 0.5–6 µg/kg/min. Titrate to effect

METABOLISM AND EXCRETION
- Hepatic metabolism
- Metabolites excreted in urine and faeces

CHEMICAL PROPERTIES
- Nil

ISOPRENALINE

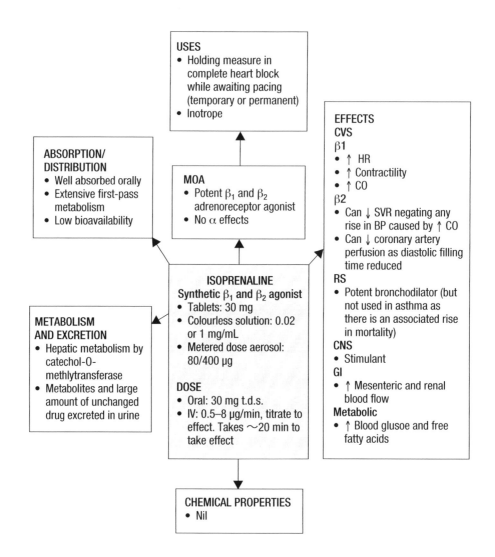

USES
- Holding measure in complete heart block while awaiting pacing (temporary or permanent)
- Inotrope

ABSORPTION/ DISTRIBUTION
- Well absorbed orally
- Extensive first-pass metabolism
- Low bioavailability

MOA
- Potent β_1 and β_2 adrenoreceptor agonist
- No α effects

EFFECTS
CVS
$\beta 1$
- ↑ HR
- ↑ Contractility
- ↑ CO
$\beta 2$
- Can ↓ SVR negating any rise in BP caused by ↑ CO
- Can ↓ coronary artery perfusion as diastolic filling time reduced
RS
- Potent bronchodilator (but not used in asthma as there is an associated rise in mortality)
CNS
- Stimulant
GI
- ↑ Mesenteric and renal blood flow
Metabolic
- ↑ Blood glusoe and free fatty acids

ISOPRENALINE
Synthetic β_1 and β_2 agonist
- Tablets: 30 mg
- Colourless solution: 0.02 or 1 mg/mL
- Metered dose aerosol: 80/400 μg

DOSE
- Oral: 30 mg t.d.s.
- IV: 0.5–8 μg/min, titrate to effect. Takes ∼20 min to take effect

METABOLISM AND EXCRETION
- Hepatic metabolism by catechol-O-methlytransferase
- Metabolites and large amount of unchanged drug excreted in urine

CHEMICAL PROPERTIES
- Nil

MILRINONE

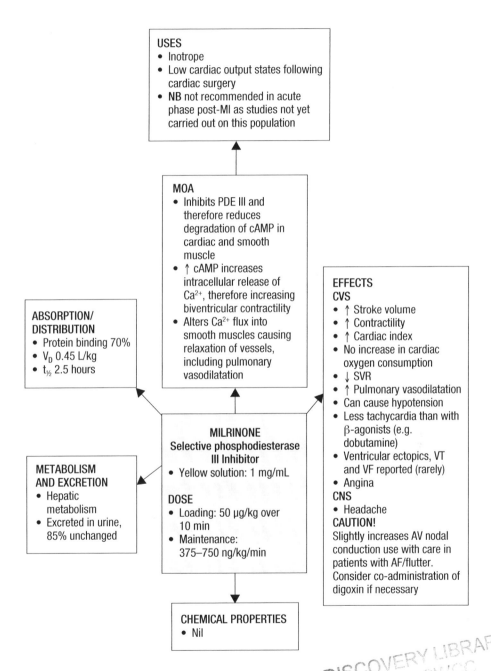

USES
- Inotrope
- Low cardiac output states following cardiac surgery
- **NB** not recommended in acute phase post-MI as studies not yet carried out on this population

MOA
- Inhibits PDE III and therefore reduces degradation of cAMP in cardiac and smooth muscle
- ↑ cAMP increases intracellular release of Ca^{2+}, therefore increasing biventricular contractility
- Alters Ca^{2+} flux into smooth muscles causing relaxation of vessels, including pulmonary vasodilatation

ABSORPTION/ DISTRIBUTION
- Protein binding 70%
- V_D 0.45 L/kg
- $t_{\frac{1}{2}}$ 2.5 hours

EFFECTS
CVS
- ↑ Stroke volume
- ↑ Contractility
- ↑ Cardiac index
- No increase in cardiac oxygen consumption
- ↓ SVR
- ↑ Pulmonary vasodilatation
- Can cause hypotension
- Less tachycardia than with β-agonists (e.g. dobutamine)
- Ventricular ectopics, VT and VF reported (rarely)
- Angina
CNS
- Headache
CAUTION!
Slightly increases AV nodal conduction use with care in patients with AF/flutter. Consider co-administration of digoxin if necessary

MILRINONE
Selective phosphodiesterase III Inhibitor
- Yellow solution: 1 mg/mL

DOSE
- Loading: 50 µg/kg over 10 min
- Maintenance: 375–750 ng/kg/min

METABOLISM AND EXCRETION
- Hepatic metabolism
- Excreted in urine, 85% unchanged

CHEMICAL PROPERTIES
- Nil

LEVOSIMENDAN

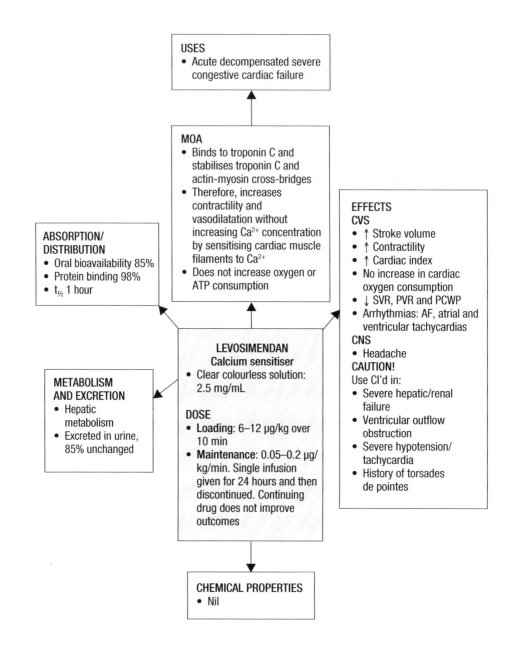

USES
- Acute decompensated severe congestive cardiac failure

MOA
- Binds to troponin C and stabilises troponin C and actin-myosin cross-bridges
- Therefore, increases contractility and vasodilatation without increasing Ca^{2+} concentration by sensitising cardiac muscle filaments to Ca^{2+}
- Does not increase oxygen or ATP consumption

ABSORPTION/ DISTRIBUTION
- Oral bioavailability 85%
- Protein binding 98%
- $t_{\frac{1}{2}}$ 1 hour

EFFECTS
CVS
- ↑ Stroke volume
- ↑ Contractility
- ↑ Cardiac index
- No increase in cardiac oxygen consumption
- ↓ SVR, PVR and PCWP
- Arrhythmias: AF, atrial and ventricular tachycardias

CNS
- Headache

CAUTION!
Use CI'd in:
- Severe hepatic/renal failure
- Ventricular outflow obstruction
- Severe hypotension/ tachycardia
- History of torsades de pointes

LEVOSIMENDAN
Calcium sensitiser
- Clear colourless solution: 2.5 mg/mL

DOSE
- **Loading**: 6–12 µg/kg over 10 min
- **Maintenance**: 0.05–0.2 µg/kg/min. Single infusion given for 24 hours and then discontinued. Continuing drug does not improve outcomes

METABOLISM AND EXCRETION
- Hepatic metabolism
- Excreted in urine, 85% unchanged

CHEMICAL PROPERTIES
- Nil

OXYTOCIN

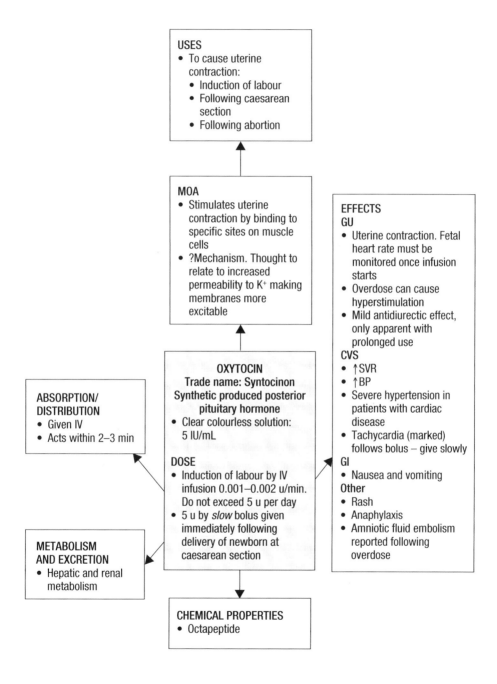

USES
- To cause uterine contraction:
  - Induction of labour
  - Following caesarean section
  - Following abortion

MOA
- Stimulates uterine contraction by binding to specific sites on muscle cells
- ?Mechanism. Thought to relate to increased permeability to K^+ making membranes more excitable

EFFECTS
GU
- Uterine contraction. Fetal heart rate must be monitored once infusion starts
- Overdose can cause hyperstimulation
- Mild antidiurectic effect, only apparent with prolonged use
CVS
- ↑SVR
- ↑BP
- Severe hypertension in patients with cardiac disease
- Tachycardia (marked) follows bolus – give slowly
GI
- Nausea and vomiting
Other
- Rash
- Anaphylaxis
- Amniotic fluid embolism reported following overdose

ABSORPTION/DISTRIBUTION
- Given IV
- Acts within 2–3 min

OXYTOCIN
Trade name: Syntocinon
Synthetic produced posterior pituitary hormone
- Clear colourless solution: 5 IU/mL

DOSE
- Induction of labour by IV infusion 0.001–0.002 u/min. Do not exceed 5 u per day
- 5 u by *slow* bolus given immediately following delivery of newborn at caesarean section

METABOLISM AND EXCRETION
- Hepatic and renal metabolism

CHEMICAL PROPERTIES
- Octapeptide

ERGOMETRINE

USES
- To cause uterine contraction and reduce bleeding:
  - Following caesarean section
  - Following abortion
- IM syntometrine used routinely following spontaneous vaginal delivery

MOA
- Stimulates uterine and vascular smooth muscle contraction? by binding to 5HT receptors
- Stimulates D_2 receptors at chemoreceptor trigger zone (CTZ) causing emesis

ABSORPTION/ DISTRIBUTION
- Acts within
  - 1 min IV
  - 5 min IM
  - 10 min PO
- Lasts 3–6 hours

ERGOMETRINE
Ergot alkaloid derivative
- Solution: 0.5 mg/mL
- Tablets: 0.5 mg
- Combined with syntocinon (syntometrine): 0.5 mg ergometrine + 5 IU syntocinon/mL for IM injection

DOSE
- 0.5 mg IM or 0.125 mg by slow IV injection. Repeat if necessary

EFFECTS
GU
- Uterine contraction follows 1 min after IV and 5 min after IM dosing
CVS
- ↑SVR and BP
- Severe hypertension. Can be harmful in patients with cardiac disease – lasts several hours
- CI in pre-eclampsia
- Bradycardia and arrhythmias (marked)
- MI reported
- Pulmonary oedema
CNS
- Headache
- Dizziness
- Tinnitus
- CVA reported
GI
- Severe nausea and vomiting

METABOLISM AND EXCRETION
- Hepatic metabolism
- Excreted in bile

CHEMICAL PROPERTIES
- Nil

CARBOPROST

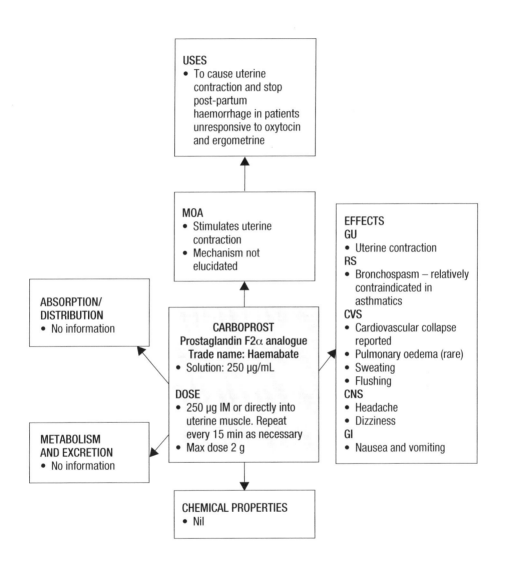

USES
- To cause uterine contraction and stop post-partum haemorrhage in patients unresponsive to oxytocin and ergometrine

MOA
- Stimulates uterine contraction
- Mechanism not elucidated

ABSORPTION/ DISTRIBUTION
- No information

CARBOPROST
Prostaglandin F2α analogue
Trade name: Haemabate
- Solution: 250 µg/mL

DOSE
- 250 µg IM or directly into uterine muscle. Repeat every 15 min as necessary
- Max dose 2 g

METABOLISM AND EXCRETION
- No information

CHEMICAL PROPERTIES
- Nil

EFFECTS
GU
- Uterine contraction
RS
- Bronchospasm – relatively contraindicated in asthmatics
CVS
- Cardiovascular collapse reported
- Pulmonary oedema (rare)
- Sweating
- Flushing
CNS
- Headache
- Dizziness
GI
- Nausea and vomiting

2

Special patient groups

CHAPTER 33

The Jehovah's Witness

Jehovah's Witnesses (JW) date back to the 1870s and consider themselves a part of the Christian religion. Their text is the 'The New World Translation' of the Bible; they believe that Jesus, the only son of Jehovah, died for our sins, but they do not accept the concept of the Holy Trinity. They maintain political neutrality, believing that only God, not government, should be in the ultimate position of authority, and consequently remain as conscientious objectors during conflict. There are, of course, many more facets to the religion beyond the scope of this book, but the one that concerns us most as doctors is the refusal of some JWs to accept transfusion of blood products. This refusal is results from the words in Genesis 9:3–4, Leviticus 17:11–12, and Acts 15:28–29.

What are Jehovah's Witnesses' beliefs surrounding transfusion of blood products?
A committed JW is forbidden, by the scriptures, from receiving blood products. Transgressing this rule compromises their relationship with God and may leave a JW feeling that life is meaningless. Giving blood products to a JW against their will has been likened, by them, to the assault of rape, in terms of its psychological impact. Each competent adult has the right to refuse to give consent to any treatment, and does not have to explain their reasons for this refusal. If a doctor wilfully transfuses a JW against their wishes, then he/she is liable to criminal and civil prosecution for assault, and also could be subject to GMC disciplinary proceedings.

Which products are unacceptable?
Unfortunately, there are no hard and fast rules, as each individual will decide which treatments are acceptable to them.

Generally, the following are not acceptable:
➤ Whole blood
➤ Packed cells
➤ White cells
➤ Platelets
➤ Fresh Frozen Plasma
➤ Autotransfusion of blood which has been taken and stored.

The individual will decide about the acceptability of the following:
➤ Blood salvage
➤ Dialysis
➤ Haemodilution
➤ Cardio-pulmonary bypass (non-blood primed circuit)
➤ Blood fractions, e.g. albumin, immunoglobulins, clotting factors
➤ Transplanted organs
➤ Epidural blood patches.

It is important to discuss beliefs with the individual before planning the anaesthetic, blood loss prevention and rescue strategies.

Patients can discuss the various blood products and strategies with a committee of elders called the 'Hospital Liaison Committee for Jehovah Witnesses'. Each hospital switchboard will have this number.

It is important to document clearly all discussions with the patient. There is a special consent form for JWs, upon which their specific individual wishes must be recorded.

How would you assess a Jehovah's Witness pre-operatively for elective surgery?

➤ A JW included on a list should be flagged up as soon as possible so that their wishes can be discussed and the best anaesthetic/surgical technique planned.
➤ A consultant who is happy to anaesthetise JWs should be allocated to the case.
➤ Clearly, the risk to the individual will be related to the nature of the surgery. It is sensible to discuss the risks with the patient alone, so that they are under no duress from other members of the church when it comes to making decisions about their treatment.
➤ The decisions made following this consultation must be entered in the notes, dated, timed and signed by both the doctor and the patient. The discussion must be frank and honest, and the consequences of refusing any blood or blood products deemed necessary impressed upon the patient.
➤ Any anaemia should be investigated and treated where possible. Oral iron may be given (this will not raise Hb acutely), or for some, recombinant erythropoietin is acceptable (though it is not licensed for this use). Discuss cases that are not straightforward with a haematologist.

How would you assess a Jehovah's Witness pre-operatively for emergency surgery?

➤ The principles of patient care are unchanged here, but there may be uncertainty as to the patient's wishes if they have lost 'capacity' by the time of presentation.
➤ Many JWs have an advanced directive detailing their wishes. If they are not carrying this, it is often lodged with their GP and efforts should be made to find it.
➤ If no advanced directive exists, or can be found, for a patient lacking capacity, we must act in the perceived best interests of the patient. This can mean giving blood/blood products if we believe the therapy to truly be life saving. The decision-making process must be documented meticulously, and a consultant must be involved in the decision.

Describe how you would conduct your anaesthetic for a Jehovah's Witness

The surgical and anaesthetic techniques must be aimed at minimising blood loss. The following options should be considered where appropriate:

➤ Arterial tourniquets
➤ Careful positioning
➤ Hypotensive anaesthesia
➤ Vasoconstrictors
➤ Haemodilution
➤ Meticulous haemostasis
➤ Optimising clotting – avoid acidosis and maintain normothermia
➤ Cell salvage, if this is acceptable to the individual and not contraindicated by their condition
➤ Drugs that promote clotting, e.g. Factor VIIa, tranexamic acid and aprotinin.

It may be sensible to stagger operations to allow for haematological recovery in between each one.

Several operations lend themselves to regional techniques, e.g. Caesarean section. This can help to reduce blood loss and also, should bleeding become life threatening, the awake patient may have the opportunity to change their mind about receiving blood/blood products.

Are there any special considerations for the post-operative period?

➤ Monitor ongoing blood loss – surgical re-exploration must not be delayed if bleeding is suspected.

➤ Patients who have suffered excessive blood loss may need to be electively ventilated in an attempt to optimise their oxygen delivery.

➤ There are reports of using hyperbaric oxygen therapy in the face of very low haemoglobins, but this is not widely available.

Issues surrounding capacity and consent

We include this section because these issues are of interest and not well covered in other texts. However, examiners will not expect you to be masters of law. To display an appreciation of the sensitive nature and potential complexity of the issues, and to show appropriate caution and seek senior advice, will be enough to pass.

Children < 16 years of age:

They may give consent if they are believed to function at a level that allows them to process the information presented to them and make an informed decision. This is called being 'Gillick-competent' and usually applies down to the age of 12 years. A 'Gillick-competent' child may consent to, or refuse, treatment. The caveat to this is that they may only refuse treatment that is deemed not to be in their best interests. In the situation of giving blood to the child, it means they may not refuse it if it is thought by the team looking after them to be life saving. Conversely, if a child who is deemed Gillick-competent consents to a blood transfusion, that consent stands even in the face of parental refusal.

If both the parents and the child refuse transfusion, or the child is not Gillick-competent to give consent in the face of parental refusal, the medical team can apply for a 'Special Issue Order' via the High Court. If granted, this will allow the doctors to give treatment. This order must only be sought in non-emergency situations where it is thought that the treatment will prevent serious permanent harm or be life saving. The manager on call for the hospital will have the procedural information for obtaining a 'Special Issue Order'.

In a life-threatening emergency, the child should be treated with whatever means necessary to preserve life, regardless of the parents' wishes.

Children 16–18 years of age:

In the eyes of the law 16–18 year olds are adults when it comes to making medical decisions. However, the parents, rather paradoxically, retain the right to consent for a child until they reach 18 years. This could lead to potential conflict if a patient aged 16–18 years were a JW but their parents were not. Here, a situation could arise in which the child refuses blood/blood products but the parents want them to be transfused. In this case, the law would suggest that the patient is treated as an adult and their choice to refuse respected, provided the patient understands the consequences of their decision. This situation has not yet been tested in the courts and therefore no precedent has been set. Looking to the law for guidance, there is no 'correct answer' to this dilemma. Whatever the decision, there are going to be serious repercussions – either the patient's wishes are ignored and medical therapy commenced or the parents' wishes are ignored and they are left bereaved. If time permitted it would be sensible to seek legal advice on such issues. All decisions must be made at consultant level.

The rights of the anaesthetist

Anaesthetists have the right to refuse to undertake elective anaesthesia on JWs but are duty bound to refer such cases to someone with the appropriate expertise, who is willing to be involved.

In emergency situations, anaesthetists are expected to provide care to JWs, and fully abide by their wishes, once these have been verified.

CHAPTER 34

Obese patient

Obesity is an increasing problem in the developed world. Consider obesity as a medical problem with associated physiological and patho-physiological consequences.

How is obesity classified?
Obesity of classified in terms of the body mass index (BMI).

BMI = weight (kg)/height (m^2)

BMI	Definition
< 18.5	Underweight
18.5–24.9	Ideal weight
25–29.9	Overweight
30–39.9	Obese
40–49.9	Morbidly obese
50–59.9	Super obese
60–69.9	Super Super obese
> 70	Hyper obese

What are the physiological changes associated with obesity that complicate anaesthesia?
➤ **Airway**
  - Higher incidence of difficult face mask ventilation and difficult intubation.
➤ **Respiratory**
  - Increased O_2 consumption and CO_2 production which may be associated with chronic hypercarbia.
  - Decreased chest wall compliance causes increased work of breathing.
  - Decreased functional residual capacity (FRC), especially when supine, means that closing capacity may encroach on FRC.
  - Increased incidence of obstructive sleep apnoea (OSA).
  - Obesity hypoventilation syndrome occurs (i.e. low O_2 saturations not caused by obstruction).
  - Increased incidence of asthma.
  - Increased incidence of pulmonary hypertension.
  These factors result in a high risk of perioperative hypoxia.
➤ **Cardiovascular**
  - Increased blood volume and cardiac output.
  - Increased incidence of ischaemic heart disease, arrhythmias, hypertension, hyperlipidaemia, heart failure and cor pulmonale.

➤ **Metabolic**
  ● Increased incidence of type 2 diabetes mellitus.
➤ **Gastrointestinal**
  ● Increased incidence of hiatus hernia, gastro-oesophageal reflux disease, fatty liver and cirrhosis.
  ● Decreased rate of stomach emptying.
  ● Raised intra-abdominal pressure which can cause compartment syndrome.
➤ **Haematology**
  ● Higher incidence of venous thromboembolism.

What are the pharmacodynamic and pharmacokinetic changes that occur?
➤ **Pharmacokinetics**
  ● Altered volume of drug distribution (V_D) and elimination.
  ● The use of 'ideal' or 'actual' body weight during drug dose calculation must be considered.
➤ **Ideal body weight**
  Height (cm) – 100 for adult males
  Height (cm) – 105 for adult females
➤ **Volatiles**
  ● Sevoflurane and desflurane – pharmacokinetics not significantly altered.
  ● Halothane – increased reductive hepatic metabolism, increasing the risk of halothane hepatitis.
➤ **Induction agents**
  ● Thiopentone – increased V_D and longer elimination half-life. Suggested dose is 7.5 mg/kg based on ideal body weight.
  ● Propofol – induction dose should be based on ideal body weight. When used for maintenance (TIVA), calculate dose using actual body weight, as propofol does not accumulate in obese patients.
➤ **Opioids**
  ● Fentanyl – pharmacokinetics not altered, use actual body weight.
  ● Morphine – accumulates in body fat, use ideal body weight.
➤ **Muscle relaxants**
  ● Suxamethonium – use actual body weight.
  ● Rocuronium – use ideal body weight.

What are the anaesthetic considerations for an obese patient presenting for surgery?
➤ **Pre-operative assessment**
  ● When planning elective surgery, pre-operative assessment should involve a multi-disciplinary team.
  ● Ensure sufficient time is allocated for the patient on the operating list. Both the anaesthetic and surgery are likely to be technically more difficult and take longer.
  ● Assess and establish co-morbidities to help define 'risk'. This will be dependent on the individual patient and the proposed surgery. The severity of symptoms, e.g. angina, may be masked by a sedentary life style. Request further investigation as appropriate, e.g. lung function tests, ECHO.
  ● Anaesthetic history, including thorough airway assessment, grade of previous intubations and patient's ability to lie flat if necessary.
  ● Consider regional techniques where possible.
  ● Optimise the patient for surgery if possible, e.g. weight loss programme and optimisation of medical conditions.

- Liaise with critical care to arrange appropriate post-operative care, e.g. HDU/ICU and non-invasive ventilation.
- Ensure a senior anaesthetist is available for the case.
- Inform theatres in advance to ensure bariatric equipment is available (e.g. electric bed, operating table, hover mattress and large blood pressure cuffs).

➤ **Induction**
- Pre-medicate with antacid prophylaxis or a proton pump inhibitor.
- If possible, get the patient to climb onto the operating table and position themselves.
- Anticipate difficult intravenous access and use ultrasound if necessary.
- Have a low threshold for invasive blood pressure monitoring, as cuffs can be inaccurate.
- Position the patient 30° head up.
- Consider awake fibre-optic intubation.
- Use a short-handle laryngoscope with a long blade and ensure the difficult airway trolley is available.
- Ensure strict preoxygenation (end-tidal oxygen > 90%).

➤ **Maintenance**
- Use short-acting anaesthetic agents, e.g. desflurane, sevoflurane, propofol, remifentanil.
- Ventilate using PEEP.
- Ensure pressure areas are padded and monitored.
- Ensure adequate fluid input given larger surface area of patient.
- Monitor and maintain temperature.

➤ **Post-operative management**
- Extubate awake and sitting up. Consider extubating onto CPAP.
- Prescribe supplementary O_2 for at least 24 hours post-operatively.
- Admit to a suitable level of care, based on your assessment of risk.
- Thromboprophylaxis.
- Multimodal analgesia.
- Early physiotherapy and mobilisation.

Obese patients are some of the most challenging patients to anaesthetise and your answer should reflect the difficulties they can present.

CHAPTER 35

Paediatric patient

Describe the physiological differences between a child and an adult
In comparison to adults, children differ in the following anatomical and physiological ways:

Respiratory system:
➤ Anatomical differences:
  • Larger head and occiput – airway best maintained with the head in neutral position.
  • Large tongue – difficult to insert laryngoscope.
  • Large, floppy epiglottis – straight blade laryngoscope typically used.
  • Narrow nasal passages and airways – prone to obstruction and fatigue as a reduction in airway radius results in a 16-fold increase in airways' resistance.
  • Flatter face profile – difficult face mask ventilation.
  • High anterior larynx (level C2/3 compared to C5/6 in the adult).
  • Narrowest point of the larynx is at the level of the cricoid cartilage (in adults it is at the laryngeal inlet) – uncuffed endotracheal tubes used traditionally to prevent tracheal necrosis due to cuff inflation.
  • Equal angles of bifurcation of left and right bronchi (in adults the right is more vertical).
➤ Physiological differences:
  • Obligate nasal breathers.
  • More compliant chest wall and horizontal ribs means breathing is more reliant on diaphragmatic rather than intercostal muscles.
  • Diaphragmatic movement is restricted by a relatively large liver.
  • Higher alveolar ventilation 100–150 mL/kg/min (60 mL/kg/min in adult).
  • Higher basal oxygen consumption 6 mL/kg/min (3.5 mL/kg/min in the adult).
  • Sinusoidal respiratory pattern, no end-expiratory pause (inspiratory: expiratory ratio 1:1).
  • Relatively fixed tidal volume, so increased minute ventilation is achieved by increasing respiratory rate.
  • Lower FRC.
  • Closing volume encroaches on FRC until the age of 5, resulting in airway closure at end-expiration (infants 'grunt' in order to maintain auto-peep to keep their airways open at the end of expiration).
  • High risk of apnoea.
  • High risk of hypoxaemia due to all the factors above.

Cardiovascular system:
➤ Circulating blood volume 85 mL/kg (70 mL/kg in adult).
➤ Haemoglobin higher in neonates 16–20 g/dL.
➤ Fetal Hb (2α 2γ) reverts to adult Hb by 6 months of age.

➤ Right ventricular mass equals left ventricular mass until 6 months of age, resulting in right axis deviation on the ECG.
➤ Transitional circulation of neonates may revert to fetal circulation if hypoxia, hypercapnia, hypothermia or acidosis occurs.
➤ Stroke volume is relatively fixed so cardiac output is largely dependent on heart rate, hence neonates cannot tolerate bradycardia.
➤ Cardiac output 200 mL/kg/min.
➤ Parasympathetic nervous system more developed than the sympathetic, hence bradycardia occurs with hypoxia or vagal stimulation.
➤ Asystolic cardiac arrest is the most common type, and mostly results from hypoxia.

Central Nervous System:
➤ Myelination is incomplete in the first year of life.
➤ Skull is not rigid because of open fontanelles.
➤ MAC infant > neonate > adult.
➤ More sensitive to opiate induced respiratory depression and apnoea.
➤ Immature neuromuscular junctions with relatively fewer nicotinic ACh receptors cause increased sensitivity to non-depolarising muscle relaxants but relative resistance to suxamethonium (dose = 1.5 mg/kg).
➤ Spinal cord ends at L3 (L1 by age 2 years).

Renal System:
➤ 80% total body water at birth (70% in adult).
➤ Increased extracelluar fluid volume causing larger volumes of distribution of drugs.
➤ Renal immaturity causes poor handling of excess water and sodium.
➤ Glucose reabsorption is limited.
➤ Glomerular filtration and tubular reabsorption is reduced until 6–8 months of age.
➤ Renal blood flow is 6% of cardiac output at birth. This rises to 18% of cardiac output at 1 month (20% in adult).
➤ Glomerular filtration rate of a term baby is approximately 30 mL/min, increasing to 110 mL/min by age 2 years.

Liver:
➤ Immature liver has fewer selective pathways by which to metabolise drugs.
➤ Low hepatic glycogen stores means hypoglycaemia occurs readily with prolonged fasting.

Temperature Homeostasis:
➤ Poor temperature regulation in neonates.
➤ Large body surface area to volume ratio.
➤ High heat loss from large heads.
➤ Higher thermoneutral temperature (i.e. the temperature below which an individual is unable to maintain core body temperature) 32°C in a term baby compared with 28°C in an adult.
➤ Infants of < 3 months of age cannot shiver.
➤ They utilise non-shivering brown fat thermogenesis.

CHAPTER 36

Pregnant patient

The changes in maternal physiology are covered in the physiology section (*Study Guide 1, Part 1, Chapter 35*). In this question we consider how these changes affect our choice of anaesthetic and why. The following refers to a pregnant patient who is undergoing non-obstetric surgery.

Which general issues should be considered when planning to anaesthetise a pregnant woman?

General anaesthesia during pregnancy is associated with an increased risk of intrauterine growth retardation, early labour and early infant death. For these reasons, elective surgery is contraindicated during pregnancy.

The following factors are of importance:

➤ There are two patients to consider, though the mother's needs must take priority.
  ● The case should be discussed with a senior anaesthetist.
  ● Surgery should be carried out by a senior surgeon who can complete the procedure in a timely fashion.
➤ The type of surgery proposed.
  ● Consider whether regional anaesthetic techniques would be appropriate.
➤ The stage of the pregnancy and its effect on maternal physiology (for details *see* answer on 'Maternal physiology in pregnancy' in *Study Guide 1, Part 1, Chapter 35*).
  ● Stomach emptying may be delayed from 12 weeks onwards, so avoid using a laryngeal mask airway beyond the first trimester; patients should be intubated.
  ● The most teratogenic period is thought to be 31–71 days. From 24 weeks onwards, the fetus may potentially survive outside the uterus.
  ● The choice of anaesthetic drugs and their potential effects on the fetus must be taken into consideration (*see* list of drug effects at end of this question).

How would you anaesthetise a woman who is 24 weeks pregnant for an appendicectomy?

➤ **Pre-operatively:**
  ● Inform the anaesthetic consultant of the patient.
  ● Confirm the diagnosis and the need for the operation with the surgeons.
  ● Consent the woman for rapid sequence induction of general anaesthesia.
➤ **Induction:**
  ● Place the table on a left lateral tilt, to reduce the risk of aorto-caval compression by the gravid uterus.
  ● Gain IV access with a large bore (≥ 16G) cannula.
  ● Have a low threshold for inserting an arterial line, both to monitor BP and also to allow regular blood gas analysis.
  ● Pre-oxygenate at 30° head up to maintain FRC.
  ● Ensure adequate pre-oxygenation as pregnant women have increased oxygen consumption and consequently desaturate more rapidly. In addition, intubation

may be more difficult because of enlarged breasts making insertion of the laryngoscope awkward.

- Induction drugs: thiopentone 5 mg/kg and suxamethonium 2 mg/kg.

➤ **Intraoperative:**

- Ventilate with oxygen, air and isoflurane. Avoid hypoxia or hypercarbia as these will alter blood flow to the placental bed. The fetus can adapt to short periods of maternal hypoxia by increasing its oxygen extraction, but in the face of long-standing hypoxia, the utero-placental bed will constrict and fetal hypoxia will result. Maternal hyperoxia is not detrimental to the fetus but maternal hypercarbia results in fetal respiratory acidosis as the CO_2 passes freely across the placenta.
- MAC falls in pregnancy, but maintain adequate end-tidal isoflurane concentration to ensure that the patient is not aware.
- Maintain relaxation with atracurium, rocuronium or vecuronium, none of which crosses the placenta in significant amounts.
- Provide analgesia with paracetamol and morphine. Do not give NSAIDs; these should be avoided in the latter stages of pregnancy as they promote closure of the ductus arteriosus.
- Give fluid, guided by clinical parameters; BP, heart rate and urine output.
- If vasopressors are needed, ephedrine has a long history of use in obstetric anaesthesia and is thought to have least effect on the placental blood flow.

➤ **Post-operatively:**

- Extubate the patient awake and sitting up. Check for an air leak with the cuff deflated to ensure no laryngeal oedema.
- Ensure sufficient analgesia; the patient must be able to cough and breathe easily to avoid chest infection, hyperventilation causing a respiratory alkalosis, or hypoventilation causing acidosis.
- Discharge to an appropriate level of care, depending on patient's condition.

THE EFFECT OF DRUGS ON THE MOTHER AND THE FETUS

At 24 weeks, the fetus is past the 'teratogenic window' (31–71 days). There are few certainties about the use of drugs in pregnancy, and although many anaesthetic agents are thought to be safe from anecdotal evidence, the manufacturers will not officially endorse their use in pregnancy.

NITROUS OXIDE	Inhibits methionine-synthase and tetrahydrofolate reductase and has been shown to be teratogenic in rats. However, this was when used at high concentration for prolonged periods. The clinical implication of this, when used for a short period of time in humans, is questionable, and certainly it provides the mainstay of analgesia during labour.
VOLATILE AGENTS	There are many conflicting studies, some showing potential teratogenicity in animals, although the design of some of these is questionable. At best, the clinical relevance of these findings is not clear. Most would advocate the use of isoflurane or sevoflurane where necessary.

THIOPENTONE	Teratogenic in high doses in animals. Causes a fall in utero-placental blood flow (up to 35%), which is not sustained. This is the intravenous induction agent of choice, and if it cannot be used, e.g. allergy, etomidate should be the next choice.
PROPOFOL	Does not alter uterine blood flow, but studies show it decreases perinatal survival and so the manufacturers advise against using in pregnancy.
NON-DEPOLARISING MUSCLE RELAXANTS	Non-teratogenic, and these bulky drugs do not cross the placenta well. Their duration of action may be prolonged, presumably due to altered hepatic metabolism. This is not true of atracurium because of Hoffman degradation.
AMIDE LOCAL ANAESTHETICS	Not teratogenic.
OPIOIDS	Considered safe in pregnancy at appropriate doses.

CHAPTER 37

Down's syndrome

Down's syndrome (DS) is one of the most common chromosomal abnormalities, occurring in approximately 1 in 700 live births. It is due to the presence of either a whole, or part of an extra 21st chromosome and is hence termed trisomy 21. In the majority of these cases the cause is due to non-disjunction of the chromosomes (95%) but it can also be due to translocation.

What are the anaesthetic considerations in a patient with Down's syndrome?
Patients with DS may have several anatomical and physiological abnormalities that can cause problems during anaesthesia and as such these cases should be discussed and performed with a consultant anaesthetist. The anaesthetic considerations are best described in terms of organ systems.
➤ **Nervous system:**
  ● Learning difficulties – these may lead to an anxious and uncooperative patient. Try to establish a rapport with the patient, tailor your explanation of the anaesthetic to their level of understanding and consider pre-medicating with an anxiolytic or sedative agent.
➤ **Respiratory system:**
  ● Atlanto-axial and atlanto-occipital instability – this is partly due to ligament laxity and can lead to spinal cord compression. Great care must be taken when positioning the head during intubation. Ask pre-operatively about symptoms of spinal cord compression and consider requesting flexion-extension views of the C-spine.
  ● Micrognathia, small mouth, macroglossia, and short neck – these may all contribute to difficulties during intubation and therefore these must be anticipated. A difficult airway trolley with appropriate emergency drugs should be ready and available. In reality, increased ligament laxity usually means that intubation is not difficult.
  ● Excessive salivation – this can obscure the view during laryngoscopy and can be an aspiration risk. Consider pre-medicating with an anti-sialogogue.
  ● Adeno-tonsillar hypertrophy and oro-pharyngeal hypotonia – all may lead to obstructive sleep apnoea. Elicit features of this condition during the pre-operative assessment (snoring, daytime somnolence, ECG evidence of right heart strain). Upper airway obstruction can worsen after anaesthesia and opioids so consider extended recovery or HDU environment in the post-operative period.
  ● Sub-glottic and tracheal stenosis – consider using a smaller than predicted endotracheal tube.
➤ **Cardiovascular system:**
  ● Congenital heart disease – occurs in up to 50% of patients with DS and common abnormalities include ASD, VSD, PDA and TOF. Apart from TOF, all of these defects cause a left-to-right shunt, which can ultimately lead to pulmonary hypertension. Full review of their medical notes with a thorough history and

examination is essential. If congenital heart disease is suspected, patients must be investigated and optimised by a cardiologist prior to surgery. Consider the need for prophylactic antibiotics at induction to prevent endocarditis.

- Difficult venepuncture – this can be due to obesity and/or learning difficulties. Consider pre-medicating patients with topical local anaesthetic agents applied to potential venepuncture sites.

➤ **Gastrointestinal system:**
- Gastro-oesophageal reflux, duodenal atresia and gastric paresis occur with increased frequency – all increase the risk of aspiration during induction of anaesthesia. Therefore consider early NGT placement, pre-medicating with prokinetic agents and antacids and/or a rapid sequence induction technique.

➤ **General:**
- Obesity
- Increased incidence of hypothyroidism
- Impaired immunity
- Increased incidence of leukaemia.

CHAPTER 38

Sickle cell anaemia

What is sickle cell anaemia?

Sickle cell anaemia, or disease, is a haemoglobinopathy with autosomal recessive inheritance. It occurs because of a point mutation on the gene coding for normal haemoglobin (HbA) on chromosome 11, which causes the substitution of valine for glutamic acid at position 6 on the β-haemoglobin chain. This results in the formation of an abnormal β-haemoglobin chain, referred to as 'HbS'.

Homozygotes (HbSS) have only abnormal haemoglobin. Heterozygotes (HbAS) are said to have 'sickle cell trait', and possess both abnormal and normal haemoglobin. The trait is carried by 25% of West Africans, 10% of Afro-Americans and also by those of East Indian, Middle Eastern and Mediterranean origin, where selective pressures of malaria have driven its inheritance. Sickle cell trait is thought to confer some protection against falciparum malaria as the parasite normally completes part of its life cycle within red blood cells. The lifespan of the red blood cells carrying HbS is reduced, and this prevents the parasite from completing its life cycle.

What do you understand by the term 'sickling'?

At low partial pressures of oxygen, deoxygenated HbS polymerises, becomes insoluble and precipitates to form elongated crystals or 'tactoids'. These cause the red blood cell to become rigid and form a 'sickle' shape.

This process increases in the presence of hypoxia, acidosis, dehydration and hypothermia. The degree of sickling is proportional to the concentration of the abnormal haemoglobin, HbS, present in the blood.

In homozygotes, HbS polymerises at PaO_2s between 5–6 kPa, and so the red blood cells of these patients sickle continuously within the venous circulation.

In heterozygotes with only 20–45% of abnormal haemoglobin, sickling occurs at much lower PaO_2 of 2–3 kPa.

Sickled blood cells increase blood viscosity, reduce flow and occlude smaller capillaries causing venous thrombosis and distal organ infarcts. They have a reduced lifespan of 10–20 days, compared to the normal 120 days. Consequently, sickle cell disease sufferers are typically anaemic (haemolytic) and jaundiced. HbS shifts the oxyhaemoglobin dissociation curve to the right.

What are the complications associated with sickle cell disease?

Patients with sickle cell trait are usually asymptomatic under normal conditions. Those with sickle cell disease can suffer multi-organ pathology associated with a life expectancy of 40–50 years. Clinical features in those with sickle cell disease only appear from 6 months of age as adult haemoglobin begins to replace fetal, which has no β chains. Homozygotes suffer periods where their disease is worse, called 'sickle cell crises'.

Sickle cell crises:

➤ **Vaso-occlusive:** Sickled cells obstruct blood flow to an organ or tissue. Most patients have infarcted their spleens by an early age and are on prophylactic lifelong penicillin. Pain control is with simple analgesia and opiates.

➤ **Sequestration:** Painful splenic enlargement results in anaemia and abdominal distension. Management is supportive.

➤ **Aplastic:** Usually triggered by infection with parvovirus B19, which arrests red cell production for 2–3 days. Reticulocyte count and Hb fall acutely. In normal individuals this is not clinically significant, but in sickle cell homozygotes who already have shortened red cell survival, it can result in life threatening anaemia.

➤ **Haemolytic:** The rate of red cell break down increases. This is rare and usually only seen in those with co-existing G6PD deficiency.

Systemic complications:

➤ **Haematological:**
  - Chronic haemolytic anaemia.
  - Crises, as above.

➤ **Respiratory:**
  - Acute chest syndrome, which manifests as pleuritic pain, cough, dyspnoea, haemoptysis and fever. Recurrent episodes can lead to pulmonary hypertension and chronic respiratory failure.

➤ **Cardiovascular:**
  - Hypertension and left ventricular hypertrophy.

➤ **Gastrointestinal:**
  - Acute sequestration syndrome in the liver or spleen.
  - Haemosiderosis, secondary to repeated transfusions.
  - Gallstones, secondary to chronic haemolysis.

➤ **Genitourinary:**
  - Haematuria.
  - Renal failure secondary to acute papillary necrosis.
  - Priapism.

➤ **Neurological Complications:**
  - Stroke.
  - Meningitis.

➤ **Immune System:**
  - Splenic infarction increases the risk of infection by encapsulated organisms including *Streptococcus pneumoniae*, *Haemophilus influenzae* and *Neisseria meningitidis*. Asplenic patients must be vaccinated against these organisms and take oral penicillin daily.

➤ **Eyes:**
  - Proliferative retinopathy.

➤ **Musculoskeletal:**
  - Deformity of skull and long bones secondary to compensatory hyperplasia.
  - Bone pain.
  - Osteomyelitis, commonly caused by *Salmonella*.
  - Avascular necrosis, most commonly affects hip joint, but other major joints may be involved.

➤ **Skin:**
  - Ulceration.

➤ **Chronic pain:**
  - Opioid tolerance.
  - Pain management issues.

Which investigations would help confirm a diagnosis of sickle cell anaemia?
➤ **FBC:**
  - ↓ Hb (6–8 g/dl).
  - ↑ Reticulocyte count (10–20%).
➤ **LFTs:**
  - ↑ Bilirubin.
➤ **Blood film:**
  - Target cells.
  - Sickled cells.
  - Howell-Jolly bodies.
➤ **Sickledex test:**
  - Sickling is induced by the addition of sodium metabisulfite to the sample.
  - This confirms only the presence of HbS but cannot differentiate between HbAS and HBSS so is only a screening test.
➤ **Electrophoresis** (definitive test)
  - Determines the type and proportion of HbS present and is therefore diagnostic.

How would you prepare for, and conduct, an anaesthetic on a patient with sickle cell disease?
➤ **Pre-operative:**
  - Involve the haematology team.
  - Assess disease severity by assessing clinical features and laboratory findings.
  - For major elective intra-cavity surgery aim for an HbS concentration of < 40% and an Hb of 10–12 g/dL. This may be achieved by exchange transfusion.
  - Cross match blood early as abnormal antibodies are caused by previous transfusions.
  - Ensure the patient is fully vaccinated and on regular penicillin and folic acid.
  - Keep nil by mouth for the minimum possible duration and prescribe intravenous fluids during this time.
  - Avoid sedatives as this can cause hypoventilation leading to respiratory acidosis and hypoxia.
➤ **Perioperative:** Standard anaesthetic techniques may be used but particular attention must be paid to the potential problems of hypoxia, hypothermia, acidosis, dehydration and pain.
  - **Oxygenation:** Pre-oxygenate patients well and maintain oxygenation with an appropriate FiO_2.
  - **Normothermia:** Use fluid warmers and warming blankets throughout the procedure and minimise shivering as this consumes a vast amount of oxygen.
  - **Avoid circulatory stasis:** Position the patient well to prevent blood stasis in dependent parts or limbs. Avoid the use of arterial tourniquets; though not absolutely contraindicated, they should be used with extreme caution. Maintain good cardiac output to prevent venous sludging. Ideally, vasopressors should be avoided.
  - **Hydration:** Give intravenous fluids to maintain hydration and prevent venous sludging.
  - **Avoid acidosis:** Ventilate to normocapnia to prevent respiratory acidosis.

- **Analgesia:** Maintain good analgesia as this reduces catecholamine surges and minimises oxygen consumption. Be aware that these patients may be opioid tolerant and therefore are likely to benefit from early review by the pain management team.
- **Intravenous regional anaesthesia** (e.g. Bier's block): Such techniques are absolutely contraindicated in sickle cell disease, because the prolonged venous stasis would result in sickling through the limb.

➤ **Post-operative:** Attention to avoiding crisis precipitants must continue into the post-operative period for both homo- and heterozygous patients.

- Homozygotes are not suitable candidates for day surgery and those undergoing intermediate to high-risk procedures should be considered for critical care post-operatively.
- Administer supplemental oxygen.
- Continue intravenous fluids until patient is eating and drinking.
- Ensure effective analgesia using multi-modal approach and involve the pain team.
- Avoid hypothermia.

CHAPTER 39

Rheumatoid arthritis

What special considerations should be made when anaesthetising a patient with rheumatoid arthritis?

Rheumatoid arthritis (RA) is a multi-system disease, which causes a symmetrical deforming inflammatory polyarthropathy. It is more common in women than men and affects approximately 2% of the population worldwide. Its extra-articular features are extensive and some are of particular importance to us as anaesthetists. It is easiest to consider the effects of the disease in systems and consequences of medication.

General:
➤ Patients are often frail and suffer chronic pain.
➤ Steroid therapy causes thinning of the skin and care must be taken when moving them or removing sticky tape as this can tear fragile skin.
➤ Patients must be carefully positioned on the operating table. Ideally, they should position themselves on the table prior to the induction of anaesthesia. Pressure areas must be closely monitored.
➤ If planning a regional block, ensure the patient is able to position themselves to allow for this.
➤ Stiffness, deformity, joint pain and lack of fine motor control may render patients unable to use devices such as patient-controlled analgesia pumps.
➤ **Musculoskeletal:**
   • Temporomandibular joint involvement may limit mouth opening.
   • Atlanto-axial subluxation (most commonly anterior subluxation) occurs in up to 25% of RA patients and may be asymptomatic. Search for signs in the history, e.g. tingling or weakness in the limbs or loss of fine motor control. Assess the patient's range of neck movement and ensure no movement outside of this range once they are anaesthetised. If there is any doubt about neck stability, cervical spine X-rays (flexion, extension and peg views) may help. A gap of > 3 mm between the odontoid peg and the arch of the atlas in lateral flexion suggests the risk of anterior subluxation. An unstable neck may need to be surgically stabilised prior to other elective surgery. If there is actual or potential subluxation, use manual in-line stabilisation when manipulating the airway, and have a low threshold to use awake fibre-optic intubation.
   • Crico-arytenoid involvement can cause hoarseness and limit airflow, causing stridor in severe cases. If this is a concern, request a pre-operative nasendoscopic assessment of the larynx by the ENT surgeons.
➤ **Cardiovascular:**
   • Pericardial effusions are uncommon and usually asymptomatic. They can rarely cause tamponade.
   • Valvular or myocardial involvement is rare. Request a transthoracic echocardiogram if complications are suspected.

➤ **Respiratory:**
  - Pleural effusions are the most common lung manifestation of the disease.
  - Rheumatoid nodules may be up to 3 cm in diameter, and can be mistaken for carcinoma.
  - Lung fibrosis is a rare complication and may be caused by the disease or by treatment with methotrexate. If respiratory abnormalities are found, consider lung function testing.
➤ **Renal:**
  - RA can cause amyloidosis which can lead to renal failure.
  - Drugs may affect the kidneys but analgesic nephropathy is rare nowadays.
➤ **Nervous system:**
  - Carpel tunnel syndrome can occur.
  - Polyneuropathy is a rare manifestation.
  - Compression of nerves at the cord or root may occur so careful positioning is important.
➤ **Haematology:**
  - Anaemia of chronic disease.
  - Anaemia secondary to gastrointestinal blood loss caused by NSAIDs use.
➤ **Eyes:**
  - Keratoconjunctivitis sicca (i.e. dry eyes).

Drugs:
➤ **Steroids:** Patients on steroid therapy may need steroid supplementation in the perioperative period.
➤ **NSAIDs:** Check a baseline renal function and, unless contraindicated, continue with NSAIDs in the post-operative period to help mobilisation.
➤ **Disease modifying anti-rheumatic drugs (DMARDs):** e.g. gold, penicillamine, and methotrexate. These can all cause immunosuppression, which may delay wound healing and increase the risk of infection. Do not stop these drugs without discussion with the patient's rheumatologist as their benefits may outweigh their risks.

Post-operative care:
➤ Continue rheumatoid medication if possible.
➤ Keep patients well hydrated and monitor renal function.
➤ Give early and regular physiotherapy, aiming for rapid return to baseline mobility.
➤ While immobile, they will need DVT prophylaxis.

ATLANTO-AXIAL SUBLUXATION
What does 'atlanto-axial subluxation' actually mean?

The Atlas is another name for the first cervical vertebra (C1). It is derived from Greek mythology, as the 'Atlas' holds up the 'globe' that is the skull. The Atlas is unique in that it has no body; instead it is fused to that of C2 below it. C2 is also known as 'the Axis'. The name 'Axis' comes from the Latin, meaning 'axle'. It is so called because it forms a pivot on which C1, which carries the head, can rotate. The odontoid peg, or dens, is a protrusion from the upper anterior surface of C2 which sticks up through where the body of C1 should be to articulate with the anterior arch of C1. This is a non-weight-bearing joint and its unique structure allows the wide range of movement of the head on the spine.

Subluxation of any joint means partial or incomplete dislocation of that joint. In this situation, the vertebrae of C1 and 2 move out of their correct positions relative to each other and therefore can impinge on the spinal cord. Obviously, cord compression at this high level can be catastrophic. Atlanto-axial subluxation occurs with increased frequency in RA because the disease causes degeneration of the bursa lying next to the transverse ligament of the atlas, causing it to weaken (this is a thick strap-like ligament which is attached to each side of the anterior arch of the atlas and loops behind the odontoid peg, holding it snugly against the arch). If this ligament becomes lax, the peg is able to move away from the anterior arch of the atlas and to move posteriorly when the neck flexes. As it does this there is a risk that it will impinge on the spinal cord. Although atlanto-axial subluxation is reasonably common on X-ray, symptoms are actually rare.

CHAPTER 40

Diabetes mellitus

What is diabetes and how is it classified?
Diabetes mellitus is an endocrine disease characterised by absolute or relative insulin deficiency and is associated with multi-system complications.

➤ **Type 1 (Insulin-dependent diabetes mellitus, IDDM)** – characterised by loss of insulin-producing beta cells of the islets of Langerhans in the pancreas, via an immune or idiopathic mechanism. IDDM usually presents in childhood and requires exogenous insulin administration to prevent ketosis. Treatment is with insulin.

➤ **Type 2 (Non insulin-dependent diabetes mellitus, NIDDM)** – characterised by insulin resistance, which may be combined with relatively reduced insulin secretion. The main risk factors include central obesity, increasing age and family history. Treatment involves increasing physical activity, reducing carbohydrate intake, weight reduction and may require oral hypoglycaemic agents such as metformin, sulphonylureas and thiazolidediones. In later stages insulin may also be necessary.

What are the complications of diabetes?
➤ **Acute complications:**
  - Diabetic ketoacidosis (DKA); more common in IDDM than NIDDM.
  - Hyperosmolar non-ketotic state (HONK); more common in NIDDM than IDDM.
  - Hypoglycaemia, usually iatrogenic resulting from excess insulin administration.
  All of the acute complications are potentially life-threatening and constitute medical emergencies.

➤ **Chronic complications:**
  - Vascular – accelerated atherosclerosis/cerebrovascular disease/coronary artery disease/hypertension/peripheral vascular disease:
  - Diabetic nephropathy – early signs of renal failure are proteinuria and elevated serum creatinine.
  - Autonomic neuropathy – postural hypotension and impaired gastric motility.
  - Peripheral neuropathy – increased risk of tissue damage and ulceration.
  - Diabetic retinopathy.
  - Infection – increased risk of post-operative wound infection.
  - Musculoskeletal – collagen glycosylation may lead to stiff joint syndrome and has been associated with a higher incidence of difficult intubation as it can affect the temporomandibular joints.

What are the anaesthetic implications of a diabetic patient presenting for surgery?
Pre-operative assessment of the diabetic patient should determine the severity of any systemic complications, assess the adequacy of blood glucose control and exclude the presence of ketoacidosis. Diabetic patients are at increased risk of perioperative complications.

Perioperative considerations:
➤ The patient will undergo a period of enforced fasting – blood glucose will need to be maintained during this period.
➤ Patients presenting for emergency surgery may be metabolically deranged, with major acid-base and electrolyte disturbances, which need correcting.
➤ Patients presenting for elective surgery should have good glycaemic control. Measure glycosylated haemoglobin (HbA_{1c}) levels, which correlate with blood glucose control in the preceding 2 months (normal < 7%).
➤ The surgical stress response will cause a rise in blood glucose intraopertively.
➤ The patient may not be allowed oral intake of fluid or nutrition for a period post-operatively, e.g. following abdominal laparotomy.

Perioperative management:
This depends on the type of diabetes and the extent of surgery. However, the overall aim in all diabetic patients is to maintain good glycaemic control throughout the perioperative period to prevent the development of metabolic complications and electrolyte disturbances.

Minor surgery for patients with IDDM:
➤ Ensure the patient is first on the list, if possible.
➤ Omit morning subcutaneous insulin if BM < 7 mmol/L.
➤ Administer half normal insulin dose if BM > 7 mmol/L.
➤ Monitor BM at least 1 hour pre-operatively, intraoperatively and 2 hourly post-operatively until eating and drinking, and 4 hourly from then on.
➤ Restart the patient's usual subcutaneous insulin dose with their first meal.

Minor surgery for patients with NIDDM:
➤ Ensure the patient is first on the list, if possible.
➤ Omit oral hypoglycaemic on the morning of surgery.
➤ Measure BM 1 hour pre-operatively. If BM > 10 mmol/L start insulin sliding scale. If BM < 10 mmol/L monitor BM intraoperatively and 2 hourly post-operatively until eating and drinking, and 4 hourly from then on. Restart oral hypoglycaemics with their first meal.

Major surgery for patients with IDDM or NIDDM:
➤ Ensure the patient is first on the list, if possible.
➤ Start a sliding scale insulin regime at least 2 hours pre-operatively, or, ideally, the night before surgery to ensure stable glycaemic control.
➤ Infuse 5% dextrose and insulin with the aim of maintaining a blood glucose of 4–7 mmol/L.
➤ Supplement potassium as required.

There remains no consensus nationally or internationally on the perioperative management of diabetic patients presenting for surgery. However, the aims of good glycaemic, metabolic and electrolyte control are universal.

CHAPTER 41

Hypertensive patient

Hypertension can be defined as a systolic blood pressure (SBP) > 140 mmHg or a diastolic blood pressure (DBP) > 90 mmHg.

Hypertension is the most common chronic disease in British primary care and almost 50% of people over the age of 65 years have hypertension. Examiners will expect a good understanding of the pathophysiology of the disorder, its anaesthetic implications and its perioperative management.

Studies have shown that untreated hypertensive patients are at significantly increased risk of end-organ damage, which may lead to stroke, myocardial infarction, heart failure, renal failure and hypertensive retinopathy.

What are the causes of hypertension?

Hypertension may be primary (essential), which accounts for 90% of patients, or secondary (10%).

Secondary causes of hypertension:
➤ Renal disease (e.g. renal artery stenosis)
➤ Endocrine disease (e.g. Conn's syndrome/phaeochromocytoma)
➤ Pregnancy-related (e.g. pre-eclampsia).

What types of medication might a hypertensive patient be taking?

In the primary care setting, basic treatment for primary hypertension may include advice about lifestyle changes such as weight reduction, increased exercise and dietary changes such as reducing salt intake.

The following classes of antihypertensive medication may also be prescribed:
➤ Diuretics, e.g. bendroflumethiazide
➤ Beta-adrenoceptor antagonists, e.g. atenolol
➤ Angiotensin-converting enzyme inhibitors, e.g. ramipril
➤ Angiotensin II inhibitors, e.g. losartan
➤ Calcium channel anatagonists, e.g. amlodipine
➤ Alpha-adrenoceptor antagonists, e.g. doxazosin
➤ Potassium channel activators, e.g. nicorandil.

Discuss the perioperative management of a hypertensive patient presenting for surgery

Pre-operative assessment:
➤ Confirm the diagnosis of hypertension and establish current treatment.
➤ Confirm the efficacy of treatment, or establish if modification of the antihypertensive regimen is required, e.g. dose alteration, drug class switch or addition.
➤ If hypertension is severe (SBP > 180 or DBP > 110), this should be treated before elective surgery. Most would cancel elective surgery at BPs higher than this, although there is little evidence to support this decision.
➤ Search for end-organ damage throughout the history, examination and investigations. It is important to establish associated co-morbidity and assess cardio-respiratory performance, e.g. exercise tolerance.

➤ Investigations may include:
  - ECG (look for left ventricular hypertrophy or strain pattern)
  - electrolytes (diuretic-induced hypokalaemia or elevated creatinine secondary to ACE inhibitors).

Pre-operative preparation: Continue all antihypertensive medications up to, and including, the morning of surgery except for ACE inhibitors, which should be omitted for 24 hours prior to surgery as they are associated with severe refractory intraoperative hypotension.

Potential intraoperative problems:
The hypertensive patient is at increased perioperative risk and the following problems may be encountered intraoperatively:
➤ Labile blood pressure – lability is more common at certain points such as induction, intubation, start of surgery, extubation and post-operatively if pain is uncontrolled.
➤ Remember that a hypertrophied left ventricle is at severe risk of perioperative sub-endocardial myocardial ischaemia. This may occur if there is a fall in coronary perfusion pressure or coronary filling time, and so low BP and tachycardia should be avoided.
➤ Vasoactive agents should be administered cautiously to hypertensive patients as the response may be exaggerated, particularly in the setting of pre-existing antihypertensive medication administration.
➤ Organs which autoregulate their blood supply (e.g. cerebral circulation) will have a right shift in the autoregulation curve, which may result in organ blood flow being severely compromised if a hypertensive patient becomes hypotensive.
➤ Left ventricular diastolic dysfunction is common in hypertensive patients. Fluid balance is extremely important, as large fluid shifts are not well tolerated; maintenance of intravascular volume is vital.

Monitoring: Invasive blood pressure monitoring with an arterial line should be used for hypertensive patients undergoing major surgery and should be considered on an individual patient basis for other types of surgery.

Post-operatively:
➤ Rebound hypertension is a common occurrence. Myocardial work is increased by such elevations in blood pressure, but care must be taken not to cause a precipitous fall in blood pressure by rapid administration of further antihypertensives, as this may lead to hypotensive ischaemia.
➤ A full assessment of the patient in the post-anaesthesia care unit should be performed, looking for potential causes of rebound hypertension (e.g. pain, hypoxia, hypercarbia, fluid overload, hypothermia). Only once these have been dealt with should cautious administration of an antihypertensive be considered.
➤ Supplemental oxygen should be considered in all hypertensive patients.

When would you cancel a hypertensive patient's operation?
This is not a straightforward question because it requires a risk-benefit analysis, focusing on the urgency of the surgery, the severity of the hypertension and individual patient factors such as the extent and severity of end-organ damage and associated co-morbidities.

You may, however, be pushed by the examiners to give examples of what types of patient you might cancel, so this list of scenarios may be a sensible guide:
➤ Severe hypertension (DBP > 115 mmHg)/Elective surgery
  - Cancel – treat for at least 1 month prior to reassessment.

➤ Moderate hypertension (DBP 100–110 mmHg)/End-organ damage/Elective surgery
- Cancel – treat for at least 1 month prior to reassessment.

➤ Moderate hypertension (DBP 100–110 mmHg)/No end-organ damage/Elective surgery
- Cancel – treat for 5–7 days then reassess

➤ Mild hypertension (DBP 90–100 mmHg)/Elective Surgery
- Consider perioperative β-blocker if not contraindicated (e.g. administered 30 min prior to surgery) and proceed.

CHAPTER 42

Chronic obstructive pulmonary disease

Chronic obstructive pulmonary disease (COPD) is characterised by an increase in expiratory airflow resistance, which results in:
➤ Increased total lung capacity (TLC)
➤ Increased residual volume (RV)
➤ Increased functional residual capacity (FRC)
➤ Reduced forced expiratory volume in 1 second (FEV_1) to FVC ratio ($< 80\%$).

The most important cause of COPD is cigarette smoking and therefore patients with COPD may also suffer from associated smoking related diseases such as ischaemic heart disease, peripheral vascular disease, cerebrovascular disease and lung cancer.

How would you assess a patient with COPD for anaesthesia?
Assessment is based on taking a relevant history, detailed clinical examination and review of investigations.

History:
➤ Establish the degree of respiratory compromise, based on:
  ● Exercise tolerance – the ability to climb two flights of stairs without stopping correlates with good cardiorespiratory reserve.
  ● Symptoms of dyspnoea – when present at rest or on minimal exertion, this indicates severe compromise.
  ● Ability to perform activities of daily living independently.
  ● Number of hospital admissions for exacerbations of COPD, and their outcome, e.g. admission to ITU.
➤ Establish current treatment regimen, e.g. bronchodilators, steroids, home oxygen.
➤ Review respiratory physician's clinic letters.
➤ Obtain a smoking history.

Examination:
➤ Ability to talk in full sentences
➤ Peripheral or central cyanosis
➤ Nicotine-stained fingernails
➤ Use of accessory respiratory muscles
➤ Evidence of right heart failure secondary to pulmonary hypertension, e.g. raised jugular venous pressure, hepatomegaly and peripheral oedema
➤ Chest examination – crackles or wheeze
➤ Ask to observe the patient walking in the ward, if appropriate.

Investigations:
Target investigations to define the extent of the disease, establish pre-operative baseline respiratory function and enable respiratory optimisation.
➤ Bloods – FBC may reveal polycythaemia from chronic hypoxaemia.
➤ ECG – may show right ventricular hypertrophy.

➤ CXR – look for hyperexpanded lung fields or the presence of bullae.
➤ ABG – on air, as a baseline.
➤ Pulmonary function tests – spirometry (reduced FEV_1: FVC ratio) and flow-volume loops.
➤ Indicators of the requirement for likely post-operative ventilation include:
   ● $FEV_1 < 1$ L
   ● FEV_1: FVC ratio $< 50\%$
   ● Baseline type 2 respiratory failure.

What are the anaesthetic implications for a patient with COPD presenting for surgery?
➤ Anaesthesia and surgery may result in a perioperative decline in respiratory function.
➤ Certain sites of surgery are particularly high-risk in terms of post-operative respiratory morbidity in COPD patients, namely thoracic and upper abdominal surgery.
➤ General anaesthesia results in a reduction in FRC (*see Study Guide 1*, Part 1, Chapter 14, 'Effects of anaesthesia on lung function').
➤ Atelectasis reduces pulmonary compliance. This may lead to intraoperative and post-operative hypoxaemia and increases the risk of barotrauma in patients requiring ventilation.
➤ Post-operative hypoventilation is common in patients with COPD, especially when opiate analgesia has been administered.
➤ Consider the level of care required post-operatively, based on the severity of COPD and the extent of planned surgery. This may range from ward-based care to level 3 ITU support.

How can a patient with COPD be optimised pre-operatively?
The process of optimisation involves establishing the extent of the disease and so the resulting risk. This allows the employment of targeted interventions to optimise the patient's condition. A detailed assessment of the patient is essential in order to be able to obtain truly informed consent. The following interventions should be made:
➤ **Smoking cessation** – if smoking is stopped at least 8 weeks prior to surgery there is a demonstrated reduction in perioperative respiratory morbidity.
➤ **Optimal medical treatment of COPD** – ensure a recent review by a respiratory physician to ensure optimal pharmacotherapy, e.g. bronchodilators, steroids and treatment of intercurrent infection.
➤ **Incentive spirometry** – has been proven to improve perioperative outcomes and should be instituted pre-operatively.
➤ **Perioperative chest physiotherapy** – to ensure maintenance of lung volumes, secretion clearance and prevention of atelectasis.
➤ **Early post-operative mobilisation**.

Regional or general anaesthesia?
This area is controversial as the evidence supporting a reduction in overall perioperative morbidity and mortality in patients with COPD undergoing surgery under regional anaesthetic techniques is mixed. However, it is clear that excellent post-operative analgesia (via regional techniques or systemic opiates) is essential for good perioperative outcomes in this patient population.

Certain types of surgery lend themselves extremely well to regional techniques, e.g. orthopaedic lower limb surgery. These operations may be performed under spinal anaesthesia, therefore avoiding the effects of general anaesthesia for the patient with COPD.

Upper abdominal and thoracic surgery also lends itself well to epidural analgesia, allowing excellent post-operative analgesia, which may reduce perioperative respiratory complications.

Summary:

To answer this question well:

➤ Define the extent of disease.

➤ Optimise the patient.

➤ Discuss the anaesthetic and surgical implications on the perioperative course of the disease.

➤ Plan for post-operative care.

CHAPTER 43

Burns and trauma

How would you assess a patient with burns who presents to A&E?

All burns victims are considered 'trauma patients' and their assessment should follow the 'Advanced Trauma Life Support' (ATLS) guidelines. Assessment and resuscitation must occur simultaneously, with appropriate emergency treatment being instigated as injuries are discovered.

History:
➤ The ATLS 'AMPLE' history is a useful mnemonic in emergency situations.
  - **A** – Allergies
  - **M** – Medication
  - **P** – Past illnesses/Pregnancy
  - **L** – Last meal
  - **E** – Events related to the injury
➤ Establish the mechanism of the burn (e.g. explosion: risk of shrapnel and blast injury; enclosed space: risk of inhalational injury; chemical burn: risk to medical team who should wear protective clothing). In children, be aware of the potential for non-accidental injury.
➤ Ask specifically about other associated injuries (e.g. patient may have jumped out of a window to escape the fire). Head injury, fractures or intra-abdominal injury are not uncommon in this cohort.
➤ Determine the time of injury, as this will guide fluid resuscitation.

Primary survey:
➤ **Airway and cervical spine control:**
  - Cervical spine fractures must be suspected so immobilise the patient using either manual in-line immobilisation or three-point fixation technique (hard collar, sand bags and tape).
  - Look for burns to the face, oedema of the lips and oropharynx, singed eyebrows and nasal hair, carbonaceous sputum and drooling. Listen for stridor, wheeze, cough or hoarseness. These features suggest inhalational injury and if present, high flow, humidified O_2 via face mask with a reservoir bag should be administered.
  - Early endotracheal intubation should be considered as airway oedema can progress rapidly. The endotracheal tube should not be cut shorter due to the risk of ongoing facial oedema.
  - If intubation is needed, call for senior assistance and have the difficult intubation trolley at hand. The patient should remain immobilised during the procedure, unless a life-threatening 'can't intubate, can't ventilate' situation arises, when the airway takes priority over everything else. If time permits and the situation is appropriate, consider an awake fibre-optic intubating technique if there is a high clinical suspicion of an unstable cervical spine fracture.
  - Suxamethonium is contraindicated from 6 hours to 2 years after a major burn

injury because of the risk of severe hyperkalaemia. There is also an increased resistance to non-depolarising neuromuscular blocking drugs mandating the need for higher doses in these patients. These effects are thought to be due to changes in the volume of drug distribution, up-regulation of nicotinic ACh receptors, sprouting of extra-junctional ACh receptors and alterations in ACh morphology.

➤ **Breathing:**
  ● Poisoning due to inhalation of carbon monoxide (CO) (generated by fires in enclosed spaces) and cyanide (generated by burning plastic) is a significant risk.
  ● Oxygen saturations recorded with a pulse oximeter will be falsely high in the presence of carboxyhaemoglobin (HbCO) and therefore a co-oximeter, which can differentiate HbCO from oxyhaemoglobin, should be used. Arterial blood gas samples should be taken.
  ● Circumferential burns to the chest can restrict ventilation and an escharotomy may be necessary. These are not usually needed within the first 6 hours of a burn.

➤ **Circulation and haemorrhage control:**
  ● Burns are associated with large fluid shifts, as fluid from the intravascular space escapes into the extracellular tissues, causing oedema. Aggressive resuscitation is required to maintain adequate cardiac output and minimise the risk of organ failure.
  ● Two large-bore 14G cannula should be sited; this may be difficult if the arms and legs are extensively burned.
  ● Circumferential burns to limbs can constrict blood supply and may require escharotomies.
  ● There are several formulae that can be used to calculate the volume for fluid replacement (e.g. Parkland, Mount Vernon and Brook formulae) but the ATLS guidelines recommend the use of the Parkland formula:

  Parkland Formula = 4 mL/kg crystalloid × % burn

  This is the total volume given over the first 24 hours: half of the total volume should be given over 8 hours, and the remaining half over 16 hours.
  For the second 24 hours fluid, administer fluid at a rate of 2 mL/kg crystalloid × % burn.
  Time is calculated from the time of the burn and not from the time of arrival into hospital.
  This formula only provides an estimate of the fluid volume required for resuscitation. In addition to this, the normal daily fluid requirements must be administered.

➤ **Neurological assessment and pain control:**
  ● GCS and pupil reactivity must be assessed as CO poisoning, hypoxia, hypotension or traumatic head injury can impair neurological function.
  ● Burns may be excruciatingly painful and therefore analgesics, including opiates, should be administered promptly.

➤ **Burn assessment and avoidance of hypothermia:**
  ● In an adult, 'Wallace's Rule of Nines' is used to estimate the body surface area (BSA) involved in the burn. The body is divided into anatomical regions that represent 9%, or multiples of 9% of the total body surface; head 9%, arms 9% each, chest and abdomen 18%, back 18% and legs 18% each. The perineum represents 1%.
  ● The BSA differs in children, where the head represents 18% of the surface area, and

the lower limbs a smaller proportion. Paediatric burns charts should be consulted to estimate the extent of the burn.

- The depth of the burn is important in assessing its severity, in wound management and in determining the ultimate cosmetic and functional results. Superficial burns (e.g. sunburn) represent damage to the epidermis. They are erythematous and painful but with no blistering and heal in 2–3 days. Partial thickness burns represent damage to the epidermis and dermis. They are painful, with blisters, and heal in 10 days. Full thickness burns represent destruction of the epidermis and dermis down to the subcutaneous fat. Hair follicles and pain receptors are lost and so the burns are white, leathery and painless. They heal slowly by wound contracture.
- Patients can become hypothermic rapidly because of impaired homeostasis, heat loss through burns and the resetting of the euthermic temperature to approximately 38.5°C. This should be minimised by increasing the ambient temperature, covering exposed areas and using fluid warmers and heated blankets.

Secondary survey:
Once the patient is stable a more detailed clinical assessment should be undertaken.

Investigations:
- **Bloods:**
  - FBC may reveal low Hb from blood loss.
  - Electrolytes may show hyperkalaemia due to rhabdomyolisis.
  - Urea and creatinine may be raised in impending or established renal failure.
- **Cross match blood:** Patients may need theatre, and blood loss during surgical debridement can be rapid, exceeding 2 mL/kg per 1% of burn treated.
- **Blood gas:**
  - CO poisoning causes hypoxia with elevated HbCO levels.
  - Cyanide poisoning causes hypoxia with a lactic acidosis and an increased anion gap.
- **ECG:** Arrhythmias can occur due to hyperkalaemia, hypoxia, hypoperfusion or acidosis.
- **Radiological trauma series:** CXR, cervical spine and pelvis.

Which generic management options should be considered in a patient with extensive burns?
Many of these will apply to any sick patient, and a systems-based approach should be used.
- **Analgesia**
- **Gastrointestinal system:**
  - Patients become hypercatabolic, requiring an increased daily calorie intake and so nasogastric feeding should be started as soon as possible.
  - Ulcer prophylaxis should be given due to the increased risk of Curling's ulcers.
- **Genito-urinary system:**
  - A urinary catheter should be inserted and hourly urine output monitored (aiming for at least 0.5 mL/kg/hr).
  - Renal function must be checked daily as there is a high risk of developing rhabdomyolisis and acute renal failure.
- **Infection:**
  - Patients are at increased risk due to loss of the protective skin barrier and generalised immunosuppression.

- Special wound dressings may be used together with topical antimicrobial agents. Prophylactic antibiotics are not used routinely.
- The patient may require tetanus immunisation.

➤ **Temperature:** Tendency to hypothermia which can have widespread effects, e.g. inhibits clotting, suppresses the immune system and impairs wound healing.

➤ **Thromboprophylaxis**

➤ **Psychological support:** Patients may require counselling and support to accept both the events causing their injuries and for the resulting disability or change in appearance.

➤ **Referral to specialist burns centre:** Criteria for transfer include partial or full thickness burns greater than 10% of BSA in extremes of ages (less than 10 years or older than 50 years), partial or full thickness burns greater than 20% of BSA in all other age groups, burns to face, hands and genitals and or significant chemical burns, electrical burns or inhalational injury.

What is the normal range of carboxyhaemoglobin in the blood?

➤ Non-smoker 0.3–2%
➤ Smoker   5–6%

What are the features of CO poisoning?

Symptoms of CO poisoning vary according to the percentage HbCO present, but no dose response relationship has been found. Levels, therefore, do not predict outcome.

0–10%	None
10–20%	Headache, malaise
30–40%	Nausea, vomiting, impaired mental ability
> 60–70%	Cardiovascular collapse and death

What is the half-life of HbCO?

➤ In air: 4–5 hrs
➤ In 100% oxygen: 1 hr
➤ In hyperbaric oxygen at 3 atmospheres: 30 min.

What are the current criteria for hyperbaric oxygen therapy?

➤ HbCO > 40%
➤ Neurological symptoms or loss of consciousness
➤ Arrhythmias or myocardial infarction
➤ Pregnancy.

CHAPTER 44

Brainstem death

Brainstem death (BSD) refers to the irreversible absence of normal brainstem functioning. In the UK brainstem death equates to human death and this is based on the concept that without brainstem function, higher cerebral activity and conscious perception is deemed impossible.

Brainstem death (BSD) refers to the irreversible absence of normal brainstem functioning.

What are the diagnostic criteria for brainstem death testing?
Before a patient can be certified as BSD, certain preconditions must be met:
➤ The patient must be in an apnoeic coma and ventilator-dependent.
➤ Irreversible brain damage of known cause must be established.
➤ Reversible causes of reduced consciousness must be identified and corrected (e.g. hypoxia, hypercapnia, hypothermia, hypotension, acid-base abnormalities, metabolic disturbances, e.g. hyponatraemia, endocrine disease, e.g. hypothyroidism, drugs, e.g. sedative agents and muscle relaxants).

Only once these preconditions have been met and at least 6 hours have elapsed since the onset of coma can formal BSD testing begin.

Who can perform BSD testing?
The test requires two doctors who have been registered for at least 5 years, one of whom should be a consultant. Neither should be a member of the organ retrieval team. Each doctor should perform one set of tests, watched by the other. The two sets of tests can be done one after the other; although many choose to wait a few hours in between sets, this is not a legal necessity. Death is legally declared after the completion of the first set of tests.

Which tests are performed?
Several cranial nerves (CN) pathways integrating within the brainstem are tested in order to establish loss of brainstem reflexes to the following:
➤ **Pupillary light reflex:**
  • Pupils must be fixed, dilated and unresponsive to light.
  • Afferent pathway via optic nerve (CN II) and efferent pathway via parasympathetic fibres carried in the oculomotor nerve (CN III).
➤ **Corneal reflex:**
  • No reaction.
  • Afferent pathway via ophthalmic branch of trigeminal nerve (CN V) and efferent pathway via facia nerve (CN VII).
➤ **Painful stimulus to the face** (e.g. supra-orbital pressure):
  • No response should be elicited.
  • Afferent pathway via trigeminal (CN V) and efferent pathway via facial nerve (CN VII).
➤ **Vestibulo-ocular reflex** (caloric test):
  • 30 mL very cold saline is injected rapidly into each external auditory meatus in an attempt to induce nystagmus. If the reflex pathway is intact, the eyes move towards

the ipsilateral ear. In the event of BSD there are no eye movements. NB examine the auditory canal before performing this test to ensure it is not blocked with wax.

- Afferent pathway is via vestibulocochlear nerve (CN VIII) and efferent pathway is via CN III and abducens nerve (CN VI).

➤ **Gag reflex:**
- No gag or cough should be elicited on stimulation of the posterior pharyngeal wall.
- Tests glossopharyngeal (CN IX) and vagus nerve (CN X).

➤ **Apnoea test:** Ventilate the patient with 100% O_2 for 10 min, to ensure normocapnia, then disconnect them from the ventilator. Insufflate O_2, using a tracheal catheter placed down the endotracheal tube, to keep oxygen saturations $\geq$ 90%. Watch for respiratory effort during this period. Allow the $PaCO_2$ to increase to 6.65 kPa before terminating the test. CO_2 rises at approximately 0.5 kPa per minute during apnoea; levels should be confirmed with a blood gas.

How will you manage the patient following brainstem testing?
If the patient is not brainstem dead, medical care should continue as before.

If the patient is brainstem dead, either:
➤ Preparations should be made to withdraw life support.
➤ If the patient is being considered for organ donation, the transplant team will co-ordinate ongoing care until organ harvesting can take place.

At all stages, it is vital that the family be kept informed of events and supported through them.

3
Critical incidents

CHAPTER 45

Anaphylaxis

Anaphylaxis is an acute, Type 1 hypersensitivity reaction caused by antigens binding to IgE immunoglobulin on mast cells and causing them to degranulate. These mast cells release 'anaphylatoxins', mainly histamine, prostaglandins and leukotrienes. It is these mediators that are responsible for the physiological effects of anaphylaxis – vasodilatation, increased capillary permeability and smooth muscle constriction.

In order to undergo an anaphylactic reaction the patient must have been previously sensitised to the antigen (in this context, a drug). However, there are increasing reports of cross-sensitivity between environmental pathogens and anaesthetic agents, especially the non-depolarising muscle relaxants such as rocuronium, meaning that a patient can undergo anaphylaxis following their first exposure to the drug.

What are the signs in an anaesthetised patient?
➤ Flushing and wheels
➤ Wheezing, bronchospasm and rising airway pressures which can make ventilation difficult
➤ Oedema of face, lips and oropharynx, which may precipitate airway obstruction. Pulmonary oedema may also develop compounding hypoxia
➤ Hypotension, which may become profound with complete circulatory collapse
➤ Tachycardia.

Differential diagnosis:
Other causes of the same symptoms must be ruled out, for example:
➤ Haemorrhage
➤ Asthma
➤ High regional block
➤ Myocardial infarction
➤ MH.

The temporal nature of events may aid diagnosis of anaphylaxis.

How would you manage a case of suspected anaphylaxis?
➤ **Immediate management:**
  • State that this is an anaesthetic emergency and that you would call for senior anaesthetic assistance.
  • Stop giving the offending drug.
  • Secure the airway and give 100% oxygen.
  • If the patient is paralysed, maintain anaesthesia using inhalational agent (volatiles are not associated with anaphylaxis).
  • Administer adrenaline 50–100 μg IV (0.5–1 mL of 1:10,000 solution).
  • Repeat this dose every minute until there is an improvement in symptoms, or deterioration to cardiac arrest, in which case move onto the advanced life support algorithm.

- Give crystalloid or colloid IV to increase circulating volume.
- If possible elevate the patient's legs to improve central blood volume.

➤ **Early management:**
- Give antihistamines – chlorpheniramine 10 mg IV
- Administer steroids – hydrocortisone 200 mg IV
- Administer regular bronchodilators if necessary
- Consider iontrope or vasopressor infusion if indicated – adrenaline or noradrenaline
- Administer bicarbonate if the patient is severely acidotic
- At 1 hour, take blood for serum tryptase levels
- Admit to ITU and leave intubated if the airway or ventilation is of concern
- Check for a cuff leak prior to extubation

Put 10 mL of blood into a plain glass tube and send straight to the laboratory where it needs to be stored at –20°C. An elevated serum tryptase level confirms mast cell degranulation and therefore anaphylaxis.

➤ **Subsequent management:**
- It is the responsibility of the anaesthetist involved in the case to refer the patient to an immunologist for further allergy testing.
- A yellow card (found in the back of the BNF) should also be completed to report the adverse reaction.
- Document events in the notes, inform the patient of events, send a letter to the GP and complete a critical incident form.

CHAPTER 46

Aspiration

Aspiration is defined as the inhalation of oropharyngeal or gastric contents into the lower airways. Inhalation can lead to aspiration pneumonitis and/or aspiration pneumonia.

Aspiration pneumonitis is an acute, chemically induced inflammation of the lung parenchyma caused by the acid in the gastric contents. The extent of the damage depends on the volume and acidity of the material inhaled. If the damage is severe following this mechanism of lung injury, it is called the Mendelson syndrome, and forms one of the diseases on the ARDS spectrum. Aspiration pneumonitis does not necessarily lead to aspiration pneumonia, and therefore antibiotic prophylaxis has now fallen from favour following simple aspiration.

Aspiration pneumonia occurs when superimposed infection follows aspiration. It is most commonly seen in patients who suffer long-term 'silent' aspiration, e.g. those with neurological problems causing decreased airway protection. However, it may occur following an acute aspiration if the inhaled material is colonised with upper airway flora, or in those patients with bowel obstruction whose gastric contents may be colonised with bacteria.

What are the risk factors for aspiration?
Factors that predispose to aspiration may be divided into patient factors and surgical factors:
➤ **Patient factors:**
  - Reduced level of consciousness – anaesthesia, intoxication, head injury
  - Full stomach – recent meal, pain, trauma, opiates, bowel obstruction, pregnancy, upper GI bleed
  - Reduced barrier pressure – pregnancy, abdominal distension, hiatus hernia, obesity
  - Anatomy – pharyngeal pouch, oesophageal strictures.
➤ **Surgical factors:**
  - Operation – gastrointestinal surgery
  - Position – lithotomy or head down.

How would you manage a case of intraoperative aspiration?
➤ **Pre-operative:** Management starts with prevention, and this begins with identifying at-risk patients, followed by implementation of risk-reduction strategies:
  - Administration of antacids – e.g. ranitidine or sodium citrate
  - Administration of prokinetic drugs – e.g. metoclopramide
  - Postponing anaesthesia for 6 hours following a meal.
➤ **Perioperative:**
  - NG tube placement and aspiration of gastric contents prior to surgery
  - Use of rapid sequence induction with cricoid pressure where appropriate
  - Positioning the patient head up where possible
➤ **Management of aspiration:**
  - Call for help
  - Suction the airway
  - Administer 100% O_2
  - If possible, place patient in the left lateral position with head down

- Intubate if necessary
- Suction down the ETT once *in situ* before giving positive pressure ventilation, if possible. Consider bronchoscopy and bronchial lavage
- CXR
- Transfer to an appropriate bed, e.g. HDU or ITU, for supportive treatment – O_2, bronchodilators and physiotherapy. In severe cases CPAP or IPPV with PEEP may be required post-operatively.
- Consider antibiotics.

Treatment with steroids has not been shown to improve outcome and so is not recommended.

➤ **Antibiotics:** Antibiotics should be considered if any aspiration pneumonitis does not resolve within 48 hours, if the patient had bowel obstruction or if they have been on regular antacids as the resulting increased pH allows colonisation of the stomach. Each hospital will have its own antibiotic policy regarding aspiration, and microbiology advice should be sought.

➤ **Starvation protocols:** Patients should be fasted for the following times:

- Food: 6 hours
- Clear fluid: 2 hours
- Breast milk: 4 hours
- Bottle formula: 6 hours
- Milk: 6 hours
- Chewing gum: 2 hours

Clear fluid: if you are able to read the typed page through the fluid, it counts as clear. More sugar-laden fluids such as cola count as food.

CHAPTER 47

Awareness

Awareness is currently one of the most common pre-operative anxieties expressed by patients for whom awareness under general anaesthesia is a terrifying experience that can result in debilitating psychological sequelae and even post-traumatic stress disorder. For the anaesthetist, it can also lead to serious consequences with medico-legal claims for awareness constituting 2% of all claims made against American anaesthetists.

What do you understand by the term awareness?
Awareness under general anaesthesia is the ability to perceive, feel or be consciously aware of one's surroundings; this may or may not be accompanied by the experience of pain. There are two types of awareness:
➤ Explicit memory (or recall). This is the intentional recollection of events with conscious perception.
➤ Implicit memory (or recall). This is the non-intentional recollection of events with subconscious perception (i.e. these patients may remember events under hypnosis).

What is the incidence of awareness?
Explicit recall associated with pain is estimated at 0.03% while explicit recall with no pain occurs more frequently with an incidence of 0.1–0.7%.

What are the risk factors associated with awareness?
➤ **Patient factors:**
  ● Obstetric patients (0.4% recall).
  ● Patients on cardiopulmonary bypass (1.0% recall).
  ● Moribund patients for emergency procedures.
  ● Patients who are unexpectedly difficult to intubate.
  ● Patients undergoing bronchoscopy.
  ● Patients with increased resistance to anaesthetic agents including those that are febrile, hyperthyroid, young, alcoholic, use recreational drugs or morbidly obese.
➤ **Anaesthetic factors:**
  ● Use of neuromuscular blocking drugs doubles the incidence of awareness.
  ● Total intravenous anaesthesia – no real-time plasma concentration of intravenous agent can be made and therefore pharmacokinetic models are relied upon to 'predict' plasma and effect site concentrations.
  ● Inadequate administration of volatile agent – MAC is the minimum alveolar concentration, at 1 atmosphere ambient pressure, required to prevent movement in 50% of subjects in response to a surgical stimulus. The definition does not encompass the concept of awareness, only movement. There is now substantial evidence to suggest a correlation between MAC and recall, with explicit recall being extremely unlikely at MAC > 1. However, MAC is influenced by a variety of factors and published data for MAC is typically quoted for healthy, unmedicated subjects. All of these factors must be taken into consideration when interpreting MAC values.

➤ **Equipment:**
- Faulty or malfunctioning equipment.
- Equipment not used or programmed correctly by the anaesthetist.

➤ **Monitoring:**
- Failure to monitor concentration of inspired and expired volatile agents and MAC.
- Failure to monitor peripheral cannula and infusion line with TIVA.
- Failure to look for clinical signs of awareness (heart rate, blood pressure, tachypnoea, sweating and lacrimation).
- Absence of clinical signs of awareness due to drugs (e.g. β-blockers will mask a tachycardia and hypertension, anti-muscarinic agents will mask sweating and tear production, opioids will mask pupillary dilation and neuromuscular blockers will mask movement and tachypnoea).

What would you do if a patient complains they were aware under general anaesthesia?
This is a serious situation with potentially devastating consequences to both the patient and anaesthetist involved.

➤ Seek advice from a consultant.
➤ Visit the patient as soon as possible with a witness (preferably a consultant).
➤ Take a full history and elicit exactly what the patient sensed and whether they were in pain.
➤ Document all conversations.
➤ Review the medical notes and anaesthetic records and try to ascertain the cause.
➤ Be sympathetic and if true awareness is suspected, apologise.
➤ Give a full explanation to the patient.
➤ Offer a follow-up appointment and psychological support.
➤ Reassure patient that this is very unlikely to happen again.
➤ Inform patient's GP, the hospital administrators and your medical defence organisation.
➤ Complete a critical incident form.
➤ Debrief with your consultant to try to determine what, if anything, could have been done differently.

CHAPTER 48

Blood transfusion error

The Blood Transfusion Task Force has issued guidelines on the process of red cell transfusion. A summary of these recommendations is as follows:

Once the decision to transfuse has been made, the following procedures should be followed to minimise the incorrect administration of red cells to the patient:

➤ The identity of the patient must be confirmed.
➤ The blood compatibility label must be checked to ensure that the blood is correct for the patient.
➤ The expiry date should be checked.
➤ The bag should be inspected to ensure integrity of the plastic casing.
➤ Removed patient identification bands must be replaced or reattached.
➤ Blood left out of a blood fridge for longer than 30 min should be transfused within 4 hours, or discarded.
➤ The details of the unit of blood transfused should be recorded on the anaesthetic chart or in the contemporaneous clinical notes.
➤ Tear-off sticky labels may facilitate this data recording.
➤ The volume of blood transfused should be recorded once administered.
➤ 100% traceability of all allogeneic blood transfused is a legal requirement following the European Blood Directive.

Failure to adhere to the above recommendations increases the chances of a transfusion error occurring. Blood transfusion error is one of the serious hazards of transfusion (SHOT). SHOT is based at the Manchester Blood Transfusion Centre and is affiliated to the Royal College of Pathologists. Among its many roles, it aims to build an evidence base of transfusion hazards and encourage UK hospitals to participate in haemovigilance. SHOT is now entering its second decade of reporting as one of the longest established haemovigilance systems in the world. Mortality from blood transfusion is low, but there is avoidable major morbidity. In 2007 there were 12 severe (anaphylactic) cases of ABO incompatible red cell transfusion, 9 arising from clinical error and 3 from laboratory error. SABRE (Serious Adverse Blood Reaction and Events) is an on-line system submission of notification and subsequent confirmation of blood-related adverse events and reactions.

What is an acute haemolytic transfusion reaction?

If blood is mistakenly administered to the wrong patient the chances of ABO incompatibility are approximately 1 in 3. The reaction is usually most severe if Group A cells are transfused to a Group O patient. Incompatible transfused cells react with the patient's own Anti-A or Anti-B antibodies or other alloantibodies (e.g. Kell/Duffy) to red cell antigens. This reaction can lead to activation of complement and cause disseminated intravascular coagulation (DIC).

Infusion of ABO incompatible blood still almost always arises from errors in labelling the sample tube or the crossmatch request form or from inadequate checks when blood is administered.

What are the symptoms and signs of a haemolytic transfusion reaction?

(In a conscious patient even a few milliliters of ABO incompatible blood may cause symptoms (agitation, pain at infusion site, flushing, abdominal, flank or substernal pain and breathlessness) within 1–2 minutes.

Signs may include pyrexia, hypotension, bleeding, haemoglobinaemia and haemoglobinuria.

In an unconscious or anaesthetised patient hypotension and uncontrollable bleeding secondary to DIC may be the only signs of an incompatible transfusion.

How would you manage an acute haemolytic transfusion reaction?

ABO incompatibility/acute haemolytic transfusion reaction is a medical emergency which requires prompt recognition and management.

If an acute haemolytic transfusion reaction is suspected, the transfusion must be stopped and urgent steps taken to confirm or exclude this possibility. The differential diagnosis must include infusion of bacterially contaminated blood.

State that this is an anaesthetic emergency and that you would call for senior anaesthetic assistance.

➤ Adopt an ABC approach.
➤ Stop the blood transfusion and administer colloid.
➤ Support respiration and circulation as necessary with supplemental oxygen, bronchodilators, volume resuscitation and consider adrenaline, vasopressors and chlorpheniramine.
➤ Check that the compatibility label of the blood unit corresponds with the patient's ID bands, blood forms and case-notes.
➤ If a mistake is discovered inform blood bank urgently since the unit of blood intended for your patient could be given out to transfuse another patient.
➤ Inform the consultant haematologist.
➤ If clinical evidence of DIC develops transfuse platelets, fresh frozen plasma and cryoprecipitate guided by clinical state and coagulation study results.
➤ If the patient requires red cell transfusion repeat crossmatch.
➤ If bacterial contamination is suspected administer broad spectrum IV antibiotics.
➤ Take 35 mL of blood for:
  ● Haematology – 5 mL EDTA tube – FBC, platelet count, direct antiglobulin test (DAT) and plasma haemoglobin
  ● 5 mL in a dry tube for repeat crossmatching
  ● 10 mL in a citrated tube – for coagulation screen (PT, APTT, Fibrinogen)
  ● Clinical chemistry – 5 mL for urea and electrolytes
➤ Take blood cultures.
➤ Return blood packs and giving set to blood bank for bacteriology.
➤ Urine dip – haemoglobinuria.
➤ ABG – metabolic acidosis and hyperkalaemia.
➤ Monitor ECG – for changes suggestive of hyperkalaemia (from haemolysis).
➤ Maintain urine output to minimise risk of acute kidney injury.
➤ Liase with critical care if indicated.
➤ Complete hospital critical incident reporting forms.

Can haemolytic reactions occur due to red cell antibodies other than ABO?

Haemolytic reactions can be caused by other red cell antibodies in the recipient's blood, including anti Rh D, Rh E, Rh C and K (Kell).

Reactions due to anti D are rare since patients generally receive Rh D compatible red cells. Reactions due to these antibodies are usually less severe than those caused by ABO incompatibility since they do not activate complement. Destruction of transfused red cells occurs mainly in the liver and spleen. The patient may experience fever, nausea and shivering.

However, the Kidd and Duffy antigens do activate complement and can cause severe intravascular haemolysis leading to cardiac and renal failure. Kidd antibodies are often difficult to find in pre-transfusion samples.

A falling haemoglobin or a rise in haemoglobin that is less than expected after transfusion together with a rise in bilirubin and a positive direct antiglobulin test indicates that red cells are being destroyed.

CHAPTER 49

Bradycardia

As soon as you are presented with a critical incident you must be thinking of the most probable causes and how you will identify and manage them. You must be systematic in your thought process so that you do not miss anything out, as this could potentially be fatal to your patient (and thus to your performance). Your answers must be confident and to the point because in a real-life situation time is of the essence.

What is the definition of bradycardia?

In an adult a bradycardia is defined as a HR < 60 bpm, but in reality you should take into consideration any rate that is inappropriately slow for that individual and haemodynamic state.

What are the causes of intraoperative bradycardia?

➤ **Hypoxia:** This is the most important cause.
➤ **Vagal stimulation:** This can be caused during eye surgery, dilation of the anus and cervix, mesenteric retraction, laparoscopy and airway manipulation.
➤ **Drugs:**
  ● Inhalational agents (enflurane and halothane > isoflurane)
  ● Opioids (fentanyl, remifentanil and morphine)
  ● Anticholinesterases (neostigmine)
  ● Muscle relaxants (vecuronium, tubocurarine and second dose of suxamethonium)
  ● Vasopressors (metaraminol and phenylephrine can cause a reflex bradycardia)
  ● β-blockers which patient may be on pre-operatively.
➤ **Neuroaxial blocks:** High spinal blockade to T1–T4 will compromise the cardiac sympathetic accelerator fibres.
➤ **Metabolic:** Hypothyroidism and hyperkalaemia.
➤ **Disease:** Ischaemic heart disease and raised intracranial pressure.
➤ **Normal:** Athletes.

How would you manage an anaesthetised patient who developed bradycardia intraoperatively?

Remember that you need to assess and resuscitate the patient simultaneously, using an ABC approach and systematically work your way from the patient back towards the anaesthetic machine so as not to miss anything. The haemodynamic consequences of the bradycardia will determine the urgency of the situation.

➤ **Immediate management:**
  ● State that this is an anaesthetic emergency and that you would call for senior anaesthetic assistance.
  ● Ask the surgeon to stop as this will eliminate any surgical vagal stimulation.
  ● Administer 100% oxygen and hand-ventilate the patient. This allows you to assess lung compliance and adequacy of ventilation.
  ● Reduce or even stop volatile agent. Check the MAC and end-tidal concentration of volatile agent.

- Administer atropine 0.6 mg (10 μg/kg) and flush. Repeat if necessary up to a maximum of 3 mg.
- Check BP and if hypotensive give fluid bolus (10 mL/kg of either crystalloid or colloid). Repeat if necessary. Bolus vasopressors agents, e.g. ephedrine, as required.

If no satisfactory response, reassess the situation starting at ABC and treat the probable cause as appropriate.

➤ **Management options in persistent bradycardia:**
- Ask for the crash trolley.
- Administer adrenaline 2–10 mcg/min of 1:10000 preparation.
- Commence transcutaneous pacing (this can be done using defibrillator chest pads with the defibrillator machine set to pacing mode at a rate of 50–60 bpm). Expert help will later be needed to arrange transvenous pacing.
- If HR < 30 with significant haemodynamic compromise commence CPR and follow ALS algorithm for asystole.
- Terminate surgery as soon as safely possible.
- Arrange transfer to ICU for further investigation, advanced monitoring and management.
- Document sequence of events in medical notes.
- Complete a critical incident form.

CHAPTER 50

Cyanosis

Cyanosis describes the blue discolouration of the skin and mucous membranes due to the presence of increased quantities of deoxygenated haemoglobin. The name is derived from the Greek word 'cyan' for blue.

Cyanosis becomes clinically evident when arterial oxygen saturations fall below approximately 85–90%; this correlates with a deoxyhaemoglobin level of at least 5 g/dL.

This answer should be read in conjunction with critical incidents on hypoxia and difficult to ventilate.

How can you classify cyanosis?
Cyanosis can be classified as central or peripheral.
➤ **Central cyanosis:**
  • Most visible in the tongue and lips
  • Commonest causes are cardio-respiratory problems, which may be acute (e.g. obstructed airway) or chronic (e.g. some types of congenital heart disease).
➤ **Peripheral cyanosis:**
  • Visible in the fingers and nail beds
  • Caused by reduced peripheral perfusion
  • May be seen in combination with central cyanosis.

What are the causes of congenital cyanotic heart disease?
Cyanosis occurs in patients with congenital heart lesions that result in a right to left shunt of blood:
➤ Tetralogy of Fallot
➤ Pulmonary stenosis or atresia with septal defect
➤ Truncus arteriosus
➤ Total anomalous pulmonary venous drainage
➤ Transposition of the great arteries.

What are the common causes of peripheral cyanosis?
➤ All of the causes of central cyanosis
➤ Cold-induced peripheral vasoconstriction
➤ Raynaud's phenomenon
➤ Low cardiac output states (e.g. cardiac failure).

In terms of relevance to anaesthesia, the most important cause of cyanosis is hypoxia, due to airway or ventilatory compromise until proved otherwise.

CHAPTER 51

Difficult to ventilate (high airway pressures)

This is a relatively common critical incident exam question. The ability to manage this event effectively in the clinical setting requires a clear systematic approach to the problem.

What factors may cause you to experience difficulty ventilating an anaesthetised patient intraoperatively?

This can be classified into patient factors and non-patient factors.

Patient factors:

➤ Reduced chest wall compliance:
  - Chest wall rigidity, malignant hyperthermia or opioids
  - Prone position
  - Obesity
  - Kyphoscoliosis
  - Raised abdominal pressures, e.g. pneumoperitoneum
  - Inadequate paralysis or patient 'fighting' ventilator.
➤ Reduced lung compliance:
  - Pneumothorax
  - Bronchospasm
  - Lobar collapse or atelectasis
  - Pulmonary oedema
  - Pulmonary fibrosis
  - Aspiration
  - ARDS.

Non-patient factors:

➤ Anaesthetic circuit:
  - Blockage, compression, kinking of tubing
  - Incorrect connection of circuit, scavenging, reservoir bag, filter, humidifier, APL valve or PEEP valve.
➤ Ventilator:
  - Excessive tidal volumes.
➤ Endotracheal tube:
  - Kinked
  - Misplaced, e.g. oesophageal or endobronchial
  - Obstructed, e.g. sputum, blood or foreign body.

Treat the identified cause, clearly document the sequence of events on the anaesthetic chart and complete a critical incident form.

How would you identify such a case?

Presentation:

➤ Difficult to ventilate
➤ Decreased compliance in reservoir bag, poor chest expansion, low minute volume

➤ High airway pressure and alarm limits reached
➤ Abnormal CO_2 trace
➤ Hypoxia
➤ Circulatory collapse.

Describe your management
State that this is an anaesthetic emergency, and that you would call for senior anaesthetic assistance.

➤ ABC approach: assess and resuscitate simultaneously.
➤ Check basic parameters: heart rate, ECG, blood pressure, oxygen saturation, E_TCO_2 trace.
➤ Hand ventilate with 100% oxygen.
➤ Ask the surgeon to stop operating until it is safe to continue.
➤ Exclude obvious causes: start at the patient (check tube position and auscultate chest) and sequentially examine from the airway back to the anaesthetic machine. Treat the cause as you discover it. Consider switching to an alternative circuit, e.g. Ambu bag.

Consider the context:
➤ Patient position: prone, Trendelenburg
➤ Pre-existing disease: asthma, obesity, ARDS
➤ Timing of event: e.g. following central venous line insertion
➤ Risk factors: allergy, bronchospasm
➤ Surgery: e.g. laparoscopy with pneumoperitoneum.

CHAPTER 52

Failed intubation

Failed intubations occur in approximately 1:2000 cases or 1:200 obstetric cases. Patients do not die from lack of intubation but from lack of ventilation and oxygenation, and all too often the anaesthetist becomes fixated on trying to intubate at the expense of resuscitating the hypoxic patient. The Difficult Airway Society (DAS) has published guidelines on how to manage 'the failed intubation' scenario. You will be expected to know these as examiners are likely to take a very harsh view of faltering knowledge in this crucial area.

What is a difficult intubation?
A difficult intubation is defined as one in which an anaesthetist with at least two years' training, using a traditional laryngoscope blade, achieves only a poor view at direct laryngoscopy (grade 3 or 4) *or* requires more than three attempts at direct laryngoscopy *or* more than 10 minutes to intubate *or* additional equipment in order to secure the airway. Difficult intubations are thought to occur in about 1 in 65 cases.

What patient factors contribute to a difficult intubation?
➤ **Congenital**, e.g. Down's, Pierre Robin, Treacher Collins and Marfan's syndromes.
➤ **Anatomical**, e.g. Morbid obesity, pregnancy, large breasts, thick, short and immobile necks, protruding teeth, beards and receding jaws.
➤ **Disease**, e.g. Morbid obesity, acromegaly, scleroderma, rheumatoid arthritis, airway malignancy and cervical spine fractures.
➤ **Acquired**, e.g. Swelling, infection, trauma and scars.

How can you predict if a patient is likely to be difficult to intubate?
Unfortunately, there is no single test that can predict all difficult intubations and despite preoperative airway evaluation, 20% of all difficult intubations are not predicted. An anaesthetic airway assessment should encompass the following:

Review the medical records and previous anaesthetic charts:
➤ **Cormack and Lehane grade:** Establish previous grade of intubation (grade 3 or 4 is considered difficult) and any airway complications.

History:
➤ **Presenting pathology:** e.g. airway malignancies are likely to be associated with a difficult airway.
➤ **Medical diseases:** e.g. rheumatoid arthritis can affect the temporomandibular joints, neck and arytenoids.
➤ **Surgery to the neck and airway:** This can distort airway anatomy.
➤ **Radiotherapy to the head and neck:** This can distort airway anatomy and cause tissues surrounding the airway to become rigid, making head extension, jaw thrust and direct laryngoscopy very difficult.
➤ **Anaesthesia:** Ask the patient whether they had any problems, such as dental damage during previous anaesthetics.

Examination:
- ➤ **General:**
  - BMI
  - Beard (often covers a small, receding chin)
  - Large breasts (makes inserting the laryngoscope difficult; consider using a short handle laryngoscope).
- ➤ **Head and neck:**
  - Scars
  - Swellings (e.g. goitre)
  - Burns or radiotherapy
  - Range of neck movement.
- ➤ **Intercisor gap:**
  - Normal should be 5 cm or 3 finger breaths (using patient's own fingers).
- ➤ **Mallampati score:**
  - Performed with patient sitting up, head in neutral position, mouth wide open and tongue protruding with no phonation.
  - Classes I–III were first described by Mallampati in 1983 and class IV was later added by Samsoon and Young in 1987. There is now also a class 0, applicable when you can visualise the epiglottis!
- ➤ **Teeth:** Protruding teeth make direct laryngoscopy difficult while the edentulous patient makes face mask ventilation difficult.
- ➤ **Tongue:** Large tongues, as seen in patients with Down's syndrome, make inserting the laryngoscope difficult and can obscure the view.
- ➤ **Jaw slide:**
  - This gives an indication of the degree of mandibular subluxation that can occur during maximal forward protrusion of the mandible.
  - It is classified as A – lower incisors lie beyond the upper incisors, B – lower incisors meet upper incisors and C – lower incisors remain behind upper incisors.
- ➤ **Thyromental distance:** This represents the gap available to displace the tongue and should be ≥ 6.5 cm.

Radiological investigations:
- ➤ CT or MRI of upper airway and neck
- ➤ X-ray of mandible and cervical spine.

Radiological features that may aid prediction of a difficult intubation include:
- ➤ Reduced distance between the occiput and spine of C1
- ➤ Reduced distance between spine of C1 and C2
- ➤ Ratio of mandibular length to posterior mandibular depth > 3.6.

Other investigations:
- ➤ **Flexible nasal endoscopy:** Typically performed by ENT surgeons. Good views of the base of the tongue and vocal cords are obtained.
- ➤ **Flow-volume loops:** Can help to differentiate between intrinsic and extrinsic causes of stridor.

What is the Wilson risk sum score?
The Wilson risk sum score is a scoring system designed to predict the difficult intubation. It comprises five risk factors each scoring between 0–2 points with a maximum total of 10 points:

Risk factor	Variable	Score
Weight	< 90 kg	0
	90–110 kg	1
	> 110 kg	2
Head & neck movement	> 90°	0
	90°	1
	< 90°	2
Jaw movement	Intercisor gap ≥ 5 cm Subluxation = A	0
	Intercisor gap < 5 cm and Subluxation = B	1
	Intercisor gap < 5 cm and Subluxation = C	2
Receding mandible	Normal	0
	Moderate	1
	Severe	2
Buck teeth	Normal	0
	Moderate	1
	Severe	2

A score of more than 2 predicts approximately 75% of difficult intubations.

What are the management options of a failed intubation?
In any failed intubation scenario there are four questions that must be addressed in order to determine the safest management option for that patient:
➤ **Can the patient be ventilated?**
  • If the patient can be ventilated this allows time for help to be summoned and intubating aids to be brought.
  • If the patient cannot be ventilated, the 'can't intubate, can't ventilate' algorithm from the DAS should be followed.
➤ **Is this a RSI or non-RSI technique?**
  Time constraints and the risk of aspiration may complicate a failed RSI intubation.
➤ **Is surgery elective or emergency?**
  • If surgery is elective, the patient should be woken up and alternative options including awake fibre-optic intubation, regional anaesthetic techniques or local anaesthetic techniques should be considered. Alternatively, surgery should be postponed.
  • If immediate surgery is essential because without it the patient would incur serious morbidity or even death, provided the patient can be adequately ventilated, the safest option of maintaining the patient's airway (e.g. LMA Proseal™) needs to be decided.
  • Remember that the examiners are asking for what *you* would do in this situation. Do not jump the gun and offer them a technique with which you are unfamiliar; tell them which technique would be safest in your hands.

➤ **Is the patient pregnant?**
- The mother's survival is paramount.
- Two situations in which surgery may be required despite failure of intubation are maternal cardiac arrest (CPR is not effective without delivery of the baby) and imminent risk of life to the mother if surgery does not proceed (e.g. massive peripartum haemorrhage).

Post-operatively:
➤ The patient should be reviewed.
➤ The exact nature of the difficult airway must be clearly documented in the anaesthetic notes with particular mention of ease of bag valve mask ventilation.
➤ The patient must be informed of this and encouraged to alert all future anaesthetists.
➤ A 'difficult airway alert' form should be completed and given to the patient and a copy sent to the GP.

DAS have published guidelines on the management of various 'failed intubation' scenarios. You must be well versed with these algorithms, as any evidence of faltering knowledge is likely to lead to a fail. These guidelines are reproduced with the permission of DAS at the end of this question.

Do you know of any national audits relating to the difficult airway?
National Audit Project 4 (NAP 4), conducted by the Royal College of Anaesthetists and DAS, commenced in September 2008 with the aim of determining the incidence of major airway complications (death, brain damage, surgical or needle cricothyroidotomy and unanticipated ICU admission related to an airway complication) within the UK. Data was collected for one year. There are two phases to this audit:
➤ Snapshot phase: Performed over a two-week period, data on the total numbers and types of anaesthetically related airway interventions were collected. This data is then extrapolated to give the number of airway interventions that are performed within the UK per annum.
➤ Data collection phase: Performed over a one-year period, the total number of major airway complications were collected, enabling the incidence of these complications to be calculated.

At the time of publishing, the results of this audit were not yet available.

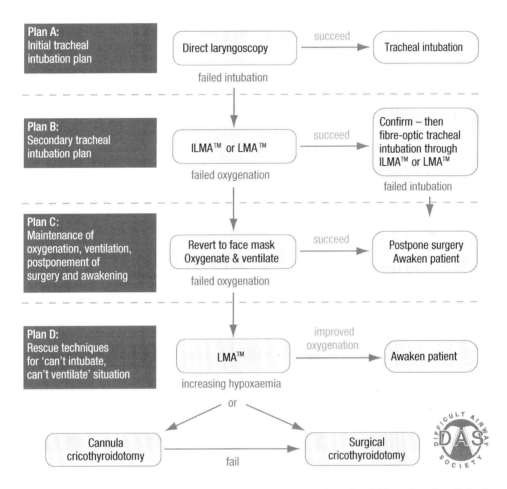

FIGURE 3.1 DAS flowchart 1 – Generic sequence of steps that should be taken in a 'failed intubation' scenario (reproduced with permission)

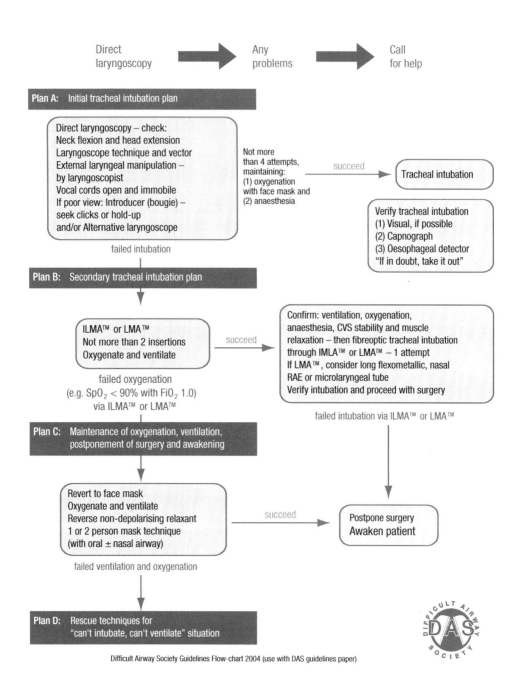

Direct laryngoscopy ➡ Any problems ➡ Call for help

Plan A: Initial tracheal intubation plan

Direct laryngoscopy – check:
Neck flexion and head extension
Laryngoscope technique and vector
External laryngeal manipulation –
by laryngoscopist
Vocal cords open and immobile
If poor view: Introducer (bougie) –
seek clicks or hold-up
and/or Alternative laryngoscope

Not more than 4 attempts, maintaining:
(1) oxygenation with face mask and
(2) anaesthesia

succeed → Tracheal intubation

Verify tracheal intubation
(1) Visual, if possible
(2) Capnograph
(3) Oesophageal detector
"If in doubt, take it out"

failed intubation

Plan B: Secondary tracheal intubation plan

ILMA™ or LMA™
Not more than 2 insertions
Oxygenate and ventilate

succeed →

Confirm: ventilation, oxygenation, anaesthesia, CVS stability and muscle relaxation – then fibreoptic tracheal intubation through IMLA™ or LMA™ – 1 attempt
If LMA™ , consider long flexometallic, nasal RAE or microlaryngeal tube
Verify intubation and proceed with surgery

failed oxygenation
(e.g. $SpO_2 < 90\%$ with FiO_2 1.0)
via ILMA™ or LMA™

failed intubation via ILMA™ or LMA™

Plan C: Maintenance of oxygenation, ventilation, postponement of surgery and awakening

Revert to face mask
Oxygenate and ventilate
Reverse non-depolarising relaxant
1 or 2 person mask technique
(with oral ± nasal airway)

succeed →

Postpone surgery
Awaken patient

failed ventilation and oxygenation

Plan D: Rescue techniques for "can't intubate, can't ventilate" situation

Difficult Airway Society Guidelines Flow-chart 2004 (use with DAS guidelines paper)

FIGURE 3.2 DAS flowchart 2 – Unanticipated difficult intubation during routine induction of anaesthesia (reproduced with permission)

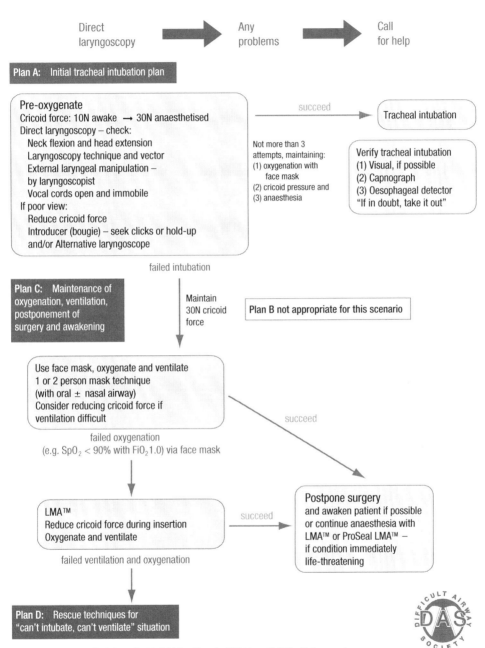

Direct laryngoscopy → Any problems → Call for help

Plan A: Initial tracheal intubation plan

Pre-oxygenate
Cricoid force: 10N awake → 30N anaesthetised
Direct laryngoscopy – check:
    Neck flexion and head extension
    Laryngoscopy technique and vector
    External laryngeal manipulation –
    by laryngoscopist
    Vocal cords open and immobile
If poor view:
    Reduce cricoid force
    Introducer (bougie) – seek clicks or hold-up
    and/or Alternative laryngoscope

succeed → Tracheal intubation

Not more than 3 attempts, maintaining:
(1) oxygenation with face mask
(2) cricoid pressure and
(3) anaesthesia

Verify tracheal intubation
(1) Visual, if possible
(2) Capnograph
(3) Oesophageal detector
"If in doubt, take it out"

failed intubation

Plan C: Maintenance of oxygenation, ventilation, postponement of surgery and awakening

Maintain 30N cricoid force

Plan B not appropriate for this scenario

Use face mask, oxygenate and ventilate
1 or 2 person mask technique
(with oral ± nasal airway)
Consider reducing cricoid force if
ventilation difficult

succeed

failed oxygenation
(e.g. SpO$_2$ < 90% with FiO$_2$ 1.0) via face mask

LMA™
Reduce cricoid force during insertion
Oxygenate and ventilate

succeed →

Postpone surgery
and awaken patient if possible
or continue anaesthesia with
LMA™ or ProSeal LMA™ –
if condition immediately
life-threatening

failed ventilation and oxygenation

Plan D: Rescue techniques for "can't intubate, can't ventilate" situation

Difficult Airway Society Guidelines Flow-chart 2004 (use with DAS guidelines paper)

FIGURE 3.3 DAS flowchart 3 – Unanticipated difficult intubation during rapid sequence induction (reproduced with permission)

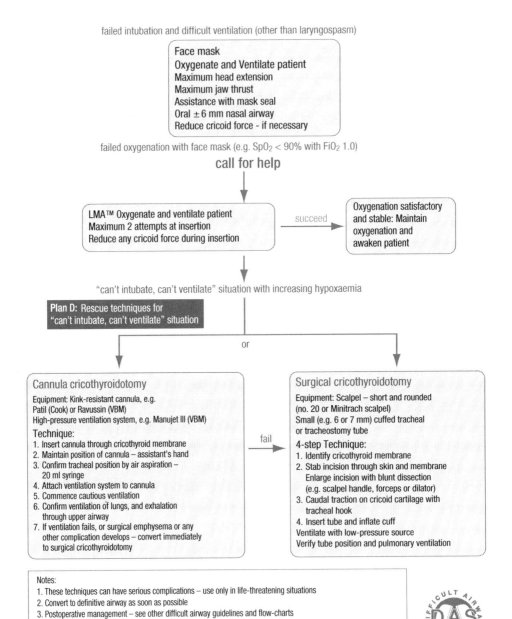

failed intubation and difficult ventilation (other than laryngospasm)

> Face mask
> Oxygenate and Ventilate patient
> Maximum head extension
> Maximum jaw thrust
> Assistance with mask seal
> Oral ± 6 mm nasal airway
> Reduce cricoid force - if necessary

failed oxygenation with face mask (e.g. SpO$_2$ < 90% with FiO$_2$ 1.0)

call for help

> LMA™ Oxygenate and ventilate patient
> Maximum 2 attempts at insertion
> Reduce any cricoid force during insertion

succeed →

> Oxygenation satisfactory
> and stable: Maintain
> oxygenation and
> awaken patient

"can't intubate, can't ventilate" situation with increasing hypoxaemia

Plan D: Rescue techniques for "can't intubate, can't ventilate" situation

or

Cannula cricothyroidotomy

Equipment: Kink-resistant cannula, e.g.
Patil (Cook) or Ravussin (VBM)
High-pressure ventilation system, e.g. Manujet III (VBM)

Technique:
1. Insert cannula through cricothyroid membrane
2. Maintain position of cannula – assistant's hand
3. Confirm tracheal position by air aspiration –
   20 ml syringe
4. Attach ventilation system to cannula
5. Commence cautious ventilation
6. Confirm ventilation of lungs, and exhalation
   through upper airway
7. If ventilation fails, or surgical emphysema or any
   other complication develops – convert immediately
   to surgical cricothyroidotomy

fail →

Surgical cricothyroidotomy

Equipment: Scalpel – short and rounded
(no. 20 or Minitrach scalpel)
Small (e.g. 6 or 7 mm) cuffed tracheal
or tracheostomy tube

4-step Technique:
1. Identify cricothyroid membrane
2. Stab incision through skin and membrane
   Enlarge incision with blunt dissection
   (e.g. scalpel handle, forceps or dilator)
3. Caudal traction on cricoid cartilage with
   tracheal hook
4. Insert tube and inflate cuff
Ventilate with low-pressure source
Verify tube position and pulmonary ventilation

Notes:
1. These techniques can have serious complications – use only in life-threatening situations
2. Convert to definitive airway as soon as possible
3. Postoperative management – see other difficult airway guidelines and flow-charts
4. 4 mm cannula with low-pressure ventilation may be successful in patient breathing spontaneously

Difficult Airway Society guidelines Flow-chart 2004 (use with DAS guidelines paper)

FIGURE 3.4 DAS flowchart 4 – Rescue techniques for the 'can't intubate, can't ventilate' scenario (reproduced with permission)

CHAPTER 53

Failure to breathe

Failure to breathe adequately following general anaesthesia requires a systematic approach to its management; the cause must be elucidated and in the interim patient's airway, oxygenation and ventilation maintained.

To establish the cause, approach the problem systematically, remembering all of the requirements for breathing, starting with the central nervous system and ending at the respiratory muscles.

What are the causes of failure to breath post-operatively?
➤ **Upper airway obstruction:**
  - Foreign body
  - Secretions
  - Oedema
  - Laryngospasm
  - Soft tissue collapse, e.g. obtunded patient or obstructive sleep apnoea
  - Vocal cord palsy.
➤ **Decreased ventilatory drive:**
  - Opiate-induced respiratory depression
  - Presence of inhalational agents
  - Extremes of arterial CO_2 tension
  - Loss of hypoxic drive in COPD patients
  - Acute intracranial catastrophe.
➤ **Inadequate respiratory muscle function:**
  - Incomplete reversal of neuromuscular blocking agents
  - Plasma cholinesterase deficiency
  - High spinal anaesthesia
  - Spinal cord lesion
  - Neuromuscular disease, e.g. myasthenia gravis
  - Restriction due to pain
  - Upper airway obstruction, e.g. foreign body, secretions, oedema, laryngospasm or vocal cord palsy.

Some of the causes of failure to breathe are examined further below:
➤ **Inadequate reversal after non-depolarising neuromuscular blockers have been administered:**
  - Signs may include uncoordinated 'see-saw' breathing movements or inability to sustain a head lift for > 5 seconds. Confirm the diagnosis by checking the patient's train-of-four with a nerve stimulator looking for fade, which would indicate a residual block. Also confirm that the correct dose of reversal has been administered.
  - Drugs administered such as magnesium sulphate can increase the duration of neuromuscular blockade.
  - Ensure that the patient is not aware during the period of inadequate reversal.

➤ **Deranged physiology:** Acidosis and hypothermia may also result in failure of adequate ventilation. Correct these where possible, and if it is not possible acutely, the patient may require a period of post-operative ventilation during which time deranged physiology can be corrected.

➤ **Poor general condition:** Malnourished patients and those with pre-existing conditions causing weakness may not have the muscle strength to sustain adequate ventilation post-operatively and again they may require a period of extended ventilation to allow recovery.

It is important to convey to the examiners a clear thought process and a structured approach to this clinical problem.

CHAPTER 54

High spinal block

Spinal anaesthesia is commonly administered to provide dense perioperative analgesia for surgical procedures involving the abdomen or lower limbs. The spread of intrathecal local anaesthetic above T4 constitutes high spinal anaesthesia.

Total spinal may be defined as intrathecal local anaesthetic induced depression of the cervical spinal cord and/or brainstem. It may occur secondary to administration of an excessive dose of local anaesthetic or excessive spread of a correct dose.

Which factors determine the intrathecal spread of local anaesthetic?
➤ **Local anaesthetic:** dosage, volume and baricity
➤ **Patient position**
➤ **Patient characteristics**, e.g. height, intra-abdominal pressure
➤ **Injection technique**, e.g. speed of injection, barbotage (i.e. repeated injection and aspiration of the fluid)

What are the clinical features of high spinal blockade?
Clinical features are determined by the height of the block:
➤ **Cardiovascular:**
  • hypotension due to vasodilatation
  • bradycardia may occur due to inhibition of cardioaccelerator fibres (T1–T4).
➤ **Respiratory:**
  • intercostal muscle paralysis leading to reduced tidal volumes
  • block above C3 will involve the diaphragm and may cause respiratory embarrassment
  • total spinal will involve the brainstem and result in apnoea.
➤ **Neurological:** total spinal anaesthesia will result in loss of consciousness.
➤ **Sensory loss:** paraesthesia in the upper limbs, may progress into the face.
➤ **Motor loss:** motor loss in the upper limbs indicates high spinal blockade.

A rapidly ascending block may present as cardio-respiratory arrest.

How would you manage a high spinal anaesthetic block?
State that this is an anaesthetic emergency and that you would call for senior anaesthetic assistance.
➤ Adopt an ABC approach. Management is supportive.
➤ Administer 100% O_2.
➤ Monitor adequacy of breathing – consider intubation and ventilaton.
➤ Support the circulation – administration of fluid plus vasopressors, e.g. phenylephrine.
➤ Treat bradycardia, e.g. atropine/ephedrine.
➤ Support ventilation and circulation until block has regressed.
➤ Document the event in the medical notes and complete a critical incident report.
➤ Inform the patient of the event.

CHAPTER 55

Hypertension

Your answer needs to be tailored to the likely cause of the hypertension, and the examiners will lead you in their questioning. Definition of what constitutes 'hypertension' in the perioperative setting is difficult. However, at the time of writing, upper limits range from 140/90 mmHg in the USA to 160/100 mmHg in the UK (*see* also Chapter 41, 'Hypertensive patient').

What are the causes of intraoperative hypertension?
➤ Patient factors:
- Pre-existing uncontrolled hypertension: essential hypertension (90% of cases), secondary hypertension due to Conn's syndrome, phaeochromocytoma or renal artery stenosis or pre-eclampsia in pregnant patients.
- Disease states exacerbated by surgery: thyroid storm or the Cushing's reflex in the head-injured patient with raised intracranial pressures.

➤ Anaesthetic factors:
- Inadequate depth of anaesthesia
- Inadequate analgesia
- Inadequate ventilation causing hypercapnia or hypoxia
- Overdosing of vasopressor drugs causing iatrogenic hypertension
- Malignant hyperpyrexia (rare).

How would you manage such a case?
➤ **Pre-operative:** An assessment should identify and optimise patient factors prior to elective surgery.
➤ **Intraoperative:** This requires an assessment to identify the cause followed by the required intervention, e.g. increase depth of anaesthesia, supplemental analgesia. Administration of antihypertensive medications may be required intraoperatively. Drugs that can be used to bring down BP in the acute setting include:
- β-blockers: Esmolol is an ultra short-acting agent given by infusion. Labetalol has α and β effects and is typically given as slow boluses titrated to effect.
- Hydralazine: A directly acting vasodilator (arteries > veins), which can be administered if β-blockers are contraindicated.
- GTN: A short-acting vasodilator (veins > arteries) and tolerance develops within 24 hours.
- Sodium nitroprusside: An arteriolar vasodilator. It is light sensitive and prolonged use can lead to cyanide accumulation.
- Remifentanil: A synthetic opioid which causes a decrease in mean arterial pressure and heart rate. Profound bradycardia can limit its use.

CHAPTER 56

Hypotension

It is hard to write a generic answer to this critical incident, as the answer you give in the exam will be tailored to the specific case presented to you. For example, it may be appropriate to discuss cardiac tamponade as a cause of hypotension in a trauma patient but it would not be appropriate as a common cause of hypotension in a 16 year old undergoing an appendicectomy.

Approach this question using the physiological formula for calculation of mean arterial pressure (MAP):

MAP = Cardiac Output × Systemic Vascular Resistance
MAP = (Heart Rate × Stroke Volume) × SVR

Thus, physiologically, hypotension may be secondary to reduced cardiac output, reduced SVR or a combination of both.

What are the causes of a low cardiac output?
➤ Bradycardia, e.g. β-blocker, opioids, vagal response, hypoxia
➤ Arrhythmias, e.g. electrolyte imbalances, valvular or ischaemic heart disease
➤ Reduced circulating volume or venous return (preload), e.g. hypovolaemia, cardiac tamponade, aorto-caval compression or tension pneumothorax
➤ Impaired myocardial contractility, e.g. ischaemia, hypoxia, acidosis
➤ Increased afterload, e.g. aortic stenosis (reduces left ventricular ejection fraction) or pulmonary embolism.

What are the causes of a low SVR?
➤ Drugs, e.g. intravenous anaesthetic induction agents, vasodilators, α receptor blockers
➤ Spinal and epidural anaesthesia, via sympathetic blockade
➤ Local mediators, e.g. potassium, nitric oxide
➤ Hypercapnia
➤ Pyrexia
➤ Sepsis
➤ Anaphylaxis.

How would you manage intraoperative hypotension?
Your management should be tailored to the likely causes. State that this is an anaesthetic emergency and that you would call for senior anaesthetic assistance.
➤ Administer 100% O_2 to maintain tissue oxygenation.
➤ Recheck measurement and ensure invasive monitoring equipment is correctly positioned relative to patient.
➤ Check what the surgeons are doing, e.g. exclude a sudden blood loss, surgical caval compression and ensure normal abdominal insufflation pressures.
➤ Correct the physiology by maintaining cardiac output and SVR which, depending on the cause of hypotension, may require any of the following interventions:

- Fluid challenge, e.g. 10 mL/kg of crystalloid or colloid. Assess response and repeat as necessary. Transfuse blood if indicated.
- Vasoconstrictors, e.g. phenylephrine, metaraminol or noradrenaline.
- Inotropes, e.g. ephedrine, dobutamine, dopexamine, milrinone.
- Treat arrhythmias, e.g. electrolyte correction, anti-arrhythmics.

If hypotension becomes resistant to treatment, consider early use of cardiac output monitoring devices to guide further therapy. Remember that even short periods of intraoperative hypotension may have consequences on end-organ function.

Decide on appropriate post-operative care in HDU or ITU if indicated.

CHAPTER 57

Hypoxia

This is an anaesthetic emergency, which requires rapid detection and management in order to prevent patient harm. Examiners will expect a well-rehearsed drill and anything less will raise serious concerns. A structured approach is required.

What is hypoxia?
➤ **Definition:** Arterial O_2 saturation < 90% or PaO_2 < 8 kPa
➤ **Detection:**
  • Pulse oximetry
  • Cyanosis occurs at SaO_2 < 85% or PaO_2 < 6.7 kPa
  • Correlates with deoxygenated Hb > 5 g/dL.
➤ **Associated:**
  • Changes in BP or changes in HR
  • Altered mental state
  • Late signs: myocardial ischaemia, arrhythmias, bradycardia, hypotension and cardiac arrest.

What are the causes of hypoxia?
➤ Low FiO_2 (hypoxic hypoxia)
  • Relative (inadequate for patient's condition)
  • Absolute (problems delivering O_2 to circuit)
➤ Inadequate alveolar minute ventilation
➤ $\dot{V}/\dot{Q}$ mismatch
➤ Anatomical shunt
➤ Anaemia (anaemic hypoxia)
➤ Low cardiac output (stagnant hypoxia)
➤ Histotoxic hypoxia (e.g. cyanide poisoning or carbon monoxide)
➤ Excess metabolic O_2 demand

Clinical causes:
➤ Inadequate alveolar minute ventilation
➤ Obstructed airway
➤ Endobronchial intubation
➤ Increased alveolar-arterial gradient
➤ Pre-existing lung disease (e.g. COPD and pulmonary fibrosis)
➤ Pneumothorax
➤ Pulmonary oedema
➤ Aspiration
➤ Atelectasis
➤ Pulmonary embolism
➤ Low cardiac output.

Prevention:
➤ Check anaesthetic machine
➤ O_2 analyser and alarms
➤ Adequate ventilation (especially tidal volume)
➤ Maintain tidal volumes in normal range
➤ Monitor and adjust FiO_2
➤ Caution with spontaneous ventilation in lung disease.

What are the causes of artificially low pulse oximeter saturation readings?
➤ Pulse oximeter malfunction – check waveform and probe position
➤ Hypothermia
➤ Poor peripheral circulation
➤ Artifacts – diathermy, motion, ambient lighting
➤ Dyes (e.g. methylene blue).

Describe your management of hypoxia
State that this is an anaesthetic emergency and that you would call for senior anaesthetic assistance.
➤ Low SpO_2 on pulse oximetry is due to hypoxaemia until proved otherwise.
➤ Increase FiO_2.
➤ Verify FiO_2 increases – check oxygen analyser.
➤ Check other vital signs – heart rate, blood pressure, ECG, end-tidal CO_2.
➤ Inform the surgeon, ask them to stop operating and to check retractors if applicable.
➤ Hand ventilate to assess lung compliance and confirm adequacy of ventilation.
➤ Check chest movements and auscultate chest.
➤ If an LMA is *in situ* consider intubation to secure the airway.
➤ Confirm endotracheal tube position and exclude endobronchial intubation.
➤ Check arterial blood gas to further define the degree of hypoxia.
➤ Verify pulse oximeter – check position, assess signal waveform and amplitude and consider changing site.

If saturations remain low, establish the cause and treat as appropriate:
➤ **Pulmonary:**
  • Pneumothorax
  • Bronchospasm
  • Lobar collapse
  • Aspiration
  • Massive atelectasis
  • Pulmonary embolism
  • Aspiration of foreign body
  • Acute pulmonary oedema.
➤ **Extra-pulmonary:**
  • Low cardiac output
  • Anaemia
  • Intracardiac shunting (e.g. congenital heart disease)
  • Histotoxic hypoxia.
➤ **Management options in persistent hypoxaemia:** Consider the use of the following interventions, the exact interventions will obviously depend upon the working clinical diagnosis.
  • Pulmonary toilet – suction endobronchial tube.

- Bronchoscopy.
- Addition of PEEP.
- Ensure adequate tidal volume 6–10 mL/kg.
- Restore circulating blood volume.
- Maintain cardiac output and Hb levels (Hb > 10 g/dL).
- Transfer patient to supine position if applicable.
- Terminate surgery as soon as safely possible.
- Optimise ventilation and decide if extubation can be achieved safely or whether a period of prolonged ventilation will be required, this will depend on diagnosis.
- Arrange check CXR.
- Arrange transfer to ICU for further management.
- Document sequence of events in patient's medical records and complete critical incident form.

CHAPTER 58

Intra-arterial injection

Inadvertent intra-arterial injection is now a relatively rare occurrence, nevertheless it remains an anaesthetic emergency requiring prompt and effective management. The consequences of intra-arterial injection depend on the characteristics of the drug injected; sodium thiopentone, for example, precipitates into crystals, which causes subsequent intense vasospasm and may lead to arterial thrombosis.

What are the risk factors for intra-arterial injection?
➤ **Patient:**
  ● Difficult intravenous access
  ● Unconscious or anaesthetised patients
➤ **Site of cannulation:**
  ● Antecubital fossa – unrecognised inadvertent cannulation of the brachial artery or aberrant ulnar artery
  ● Dorsum of the hand – inadvertent cannulation of superficial branches of the radial artery.

How would you recognise inadvertent intra-arterial injection?
➤ Awake patients will complain of pain on injection, which should always be taken seriously. Intra-arterial injection may be associated with other signs such as skin blanching leading to cyanosis secondary to arterial spasm.
➤ Severe ischaemia from vasospasm and intra-arterial thrombosis may lead to digital necrosis.

How would you manage an inadvertent intra-arterial injection?
State that this is an anaesthetic emergency and that you would call for senior anaesthetic assistance.
➤ Stop injecting the drug.
➤ Aims are to dilute the drug, dilate the artery, prevent thrombosis and provide analgesia.
➤ Leave the cannula *in situ*.
➤ Dilute the drug by flushing the cannula with 0.9% NaCl or heparinised saline.
➤ Vasodilate the artery by administering papaverine 40–80 mg if available.
➤ Administer 1000 IU heparin to minimise thrombosis risk.
➤ 10 mL 1% lignocaine will provide some analgesia and has vasodilator properties.
➤ Sympathetic blockade of the upper limb will provide both analgesia and vasodilatation.
  ● Sympathectomy may be achieved via stellate ganglion block, interscalene block or axillary block.
  ● Guanethedine block is also an option if expertise is available, and has the advantage of long-lasting therapeutic effect.
➤ Anticoagulation should be continued for 10–14 days.
➤ Consult with a vascular surgeon if necessary.
➤ Inform the patient, complete a critical incident report form and document in the medical notes the sequence of events and management.

CHAPTER 59

Laryngospasm

Laryngospasm is the reflex adduction of the vocal cords and occurs most commonly during lighter planes of anaesthesia. Direct or indirect stimulation of the larynx may precipitate laryngospasm:

➤ Direct stimulation, e.g. blood, mucus, laryngoscope or endotracheal tube.
➤ Indirect stimulation via another site, e.g. pain, cervical or anal stimulation.

Laryngospasm may present as intraoperative stridor or sudden difficulty in ventilating the patient.

Left unchecked laryngospasm may result in:

➤ Complete upper airways obstruction
➤ Desaturation and hypoxaemia
➤ Negative-pressure pulmonary oedema

What are the risk factors for laryngospasm?

➤ Pre-existing upper respiratory tract infection ('irritable airway')
➤ Smoking
➤ Children are more susceptible than adults
➤ Inadequate depth of anaesthesia for either airway manipulation or for surgical stimulus
➤ Soiling of the vocal cords, e.g. blood.

How would you manage a case of laryngospasm?

State that this is an anaesthetic emergency and that you would call for senior anaesthetic assistance.

➤ Remove the stimulus.
➤ Apply 100% O_2.
➤ Apply positive pressure to the airway to assist inspiration.
➤ If the above measures fail, deepen anaesthesia rapidly, e.g. administer a bolus of propofol at a dose appropriate to the patient.
➤ If deepening of anaesthesia fails, administer 0.15–0.30 mg/kg of suxamethonium to relax the vocal cords.
➤ Reintubation may be necessary. This will depend on the situation, patient and operation. Remember that laryngospasm may recur on re-extubation.
➤ Ensure documentation of the event and completion of a critical incident form.

CHAPTER 60

Local anaesthetic toxicity

Over the last decade there have been significant improvements in the delivery of regional anaesthesia including ultrasound-guided nerve blockade, allowing accurate delivery of local anaesthetics, and the introduction of less cardiotoxic local anaesthetics such as levobupivicaine and ropivicaine. Nevertheless, local anaesthetic (LA) toxicity remains an ever-present risk and as such, the emergency management is a core topic. The AAGBI have produced guidelines for the management of severe local anaesthetic toxicity, and examiners will expect a clear and concise reproduction of these guidelines in an exam situation.

Overview
Factors to consider in the development of LA toxicity include the LA itself, site of injection, speed of absorption and consequent rate of rise in plasma concentration. The physiological and metabolic state of the patient also may play a role, e.g. hypoxia, hypercarbia and acidosis all potentiate cardiotoxicity.

For all these reasons, the actual maximum recommended doses of LA need to be interpreted in the correct clinical context; however, examiners would expect you to know the recommended maximum doses:

LA	Max Dose	With added vasoconstrictor
Lignocaine	3 mg/kg	7 mg/kg (adrenaline)
Bupivacaine	2 mg/kg	–
Levobupivacaine	2 mg/kg	–
Ropivacaine	3 mg/kg	–
Cocaine	3 mg/kg	–
Amethocaine	1.5 mg/kg	–
Prilocaine	6 mg/kg	8 mg/kg (felypressin)

Clinical features of LA toxicity
Clinical features depend on plasma concentration of LA. For example, early symptoms in an awake patient with a plasma lignocaine concentration of 2–4 μg/mL may include light-headedness, tinnitus, circumoral tingling and tongue numbness. Plasma levels between 5–10 μg/mL will lead to visual disturbances, agitation and muscular twitching. Plasma levels above 10 μg/mL may lead to tonic-clonic convulsions followed by coma and respiratory arrest. At plasma levels of 15–25 μg/mL cardiotoxicity will result, leading to cardiovascular collapse and development of malignant arrhythmias (conduction blocks, ventricular tachyarrhythmias and asystole).

Management
State that this is an anaesthetic emergency and that you would call for senior anaesthetic assistance.

➤ Stop injecting the LA.

➤ Maintain and, if necessary, secure the airway with a cuffed endotracheal tube.
➤ Administer 100% oxygen and ensure adequate lung ventilation (hyperventilation may be of benefit by increasing pH).
➤ Confirm or establish IV access.
➤ Control seizures using a benzodiazepine (e.g. lorazepam) or use small incremental doses of thiopentone or propofol.
➤ Assess cardiovascular status throughout. Arterial line insertion would be of benefit.

Management of cardiac arrest

➤ Commence CPR following ALS protocols.
➤ Manage arrhythmias using same ALS protocols, recognising that arrhythmias may be refractory to treatment and prolonged resuscitation (several hours) may be necessary.
➤ It may be appropriate to consider other treatment options:
  • Consider cardiopulmonary bypass if available.
  • Consider treatment with lipid emulsion.

Treatment of cardiac arrest with lipid emulsion

Approximate doses for a 70 kg patient are given in italics:
➤ Administer an intravenous bolus of Intralipid® 20% (1.5 mL/kg) over 1 min (*100 mL bolus*).
➤ Continue CPR.
➤ Start an infusion of Intralipid® 20% at 0.25 mL/kg/min (*400 mL over 20 min*).
➤ Repeat the bolus injection (*100 mL*) of Intralipid® 20% twice at 5 min intervals if an adequate circulation has not been restored.
➤ After another 5 min, increase the rate of the infusion to 0.5 mL/kg/min if an adequate circulation has not been restored (*400 mL over 10 min*).
➤ Continue infusion until a stable and adequate circulation has been restored.

Remember

➤ Continue CPR throughout treatment with lipid emulsion.
➤ Recovery from LA induced cardiac arrest may take > 1 hour.
➤ Propofol is not a suitable substitute for Intralipid® 20%.
➤ Replace your supply of Intralipid® 20% after use.

Follow-up action

➤ Inform the patient of the event, answer any questions and ensure medical documentation is complete.
➤ Complete a local hospital critical incident form.
➤ Report case to the National Patient Safety Agency (NPSA) (via www.npsa.nhs.uk).
➤ Report cases to the LipidRescue™ site: www.lipidrescue.org.uk.

CHAPTER 61

Malignant hyperpyrexia

It is safe to say that the majority of us are unlikely to ever experience a case of malignant hyperpyrexia (MH) during our careers. However, malignant hyperpyrexia remains a life-threatening anaesthetic emergency with a mortality rate of approximately 10%.

Pathophysiology of MH
➤ Malignant hyperpyrexia (or malignant hyperthermia) is an autosomal dominant disorder of skeletal muscle. Its genetics are complex, with over 15 causative mutations; chromosome 19 is most commonly involved. The incidence of genetic susceptibility is now thought to be between 1:5000 and 1:10000.
➤ The various gene mutations affect the calcium release channels in the sarcoplasmic reticulum (SR). The ryanodine receptor (a calcium release channel) fails and intracellular calcium levels increase up to 500-fold, leading to sustained muscle contraction.
➤ MH is an anaesthetic-related disorder. All inhalational agents and depolarising muscle relaxants can trigger the abnormal handling of calcium within skeletal muscles.

Recognition of MH
The successful management of MH begins with its prompt recognition. MH presents in two main ways, either with excessive muscle rigidity or with signs of hypermetabolism.
➤ **Excessive muscle rigidity:** This often presents at induction as masseter spasm following suxamethonium, although generalised muscle rigidity may also occur. With ongoing muscle rigidity rhabdomyolysis occurs, serum potassium (K^+) increases (potentially causing arrhythmias), creatinine kinase (CK) increases and acute renal failure can ensue.
➤ **Hypermetabolism:** This occurs due to the increased ATP demand required to fuel the abnormal contractions and membrane calcium pumps. The earliest signs include:
  • unexplained tachycardia
  • tachypnoea (in a spontaneously breathing patient)
  • rising end-tidal CO_2 (E_TCO_2)
  • falling arterial O_2 tensions (PaO_2).
  With time, the patient's temperature rises, sometimes by as much as 1°C every 10 minutes. As more oxygen is consumed hypoxaemia and cyanosis occur, giving rise to a metabolic acidosis. As CO_2 levels continue to rise, a respiratory acidosis develops.

Management of MH
State that this is an anaesthetic emergency.
➤ Call for senior help urgently and inform the theatre team that you have an emergency. Also, call for help from any free operating department practitioners (ODPs).
➤ Disconnect patient from the anaesthetic machine immediately and begin hand hyperventilation with 100% oxygen (to reduce $PaCO_2$). Use O_2 drawn from an alternative source to the anaesthetic machine so that it is free of inhalational agents. Using a new circuit, use high flows to wash out the inhalational agents and CO_2.

➤ Maintain anaesthesia using intravenous agents (e.g. propofol).
➤ Ask an ODP to bring and prepare the 'vapour-free' anaesthetic machine for use (every department should have one and you must know where it is kept). Ventilate with this when ready.
➤ Send assistants to prepare dantrolene sodium urgently. Each vial contains 20 mg dantrolene and 3 g mannitol and this crystalline mixture must be mixed with 60 mL of water. When it is ready, give 1 mg/kg IV. Repeat dose every 5 to 10 min until the tachycardia, hypercapnia and temperature start to subside. On average 3 mg/kg is needed but up to 10 mg/kg may be required. Doses may need to be repeated in the subsequent 48 hours if the reaction recurs, though this is rare. Dantrolene works within skeletal muscles by preventing the release of calcium from the sarcoplasmic reticulum.
➤ Ask the surgeons to conclude surgery as fast as possible.
➤ Instigate active cooling measures. The surgeons are well placed to do this. Use cold intravenous fluids, cold body cavity lavages, ice packs to groin and axillae and cooling blankets.
➤ Appoint someone to record observations, drug doses, times etc.
➤ Gain sufficient intravenous access, site an arterial cannula, temperature probe and urinary catheter.
➤ Manage hyperkalaemia and acidosis expectantly, guided by regular arterial blood gas analysis and electrolyte measurements. Use insulin/dextrose and bicarbonate infusions as appropriate.
➤ Send regular clotting profiles to check for disseminated intravascular coagulopathy (DIC) and treat appropriately (e.g. with fresh frozen plasma).
➤ Manage rhabdomyolysis expectantly guided by renal function, CK levels and urinary myoglobin concentrations. Maintain urine output at 2 mL/kg/hr with fluid and diuretics to limit renal tubular damage.
➤ Finally, when stable, transfer patient to ITU.
➤ Help
  Oxygen
  Stop inhalational agents/Stop surgery
  Propofol infusion
  Intravenous dantrolene
  Temperature regulation
  Address metabolic derangement
  Liaise with ITU

Subsequent management
➤ Counsel the patient and their relatives about events and the implications of a potential diagnosis of MH.
➤ Documents events in clinical notes and inform the GP.
➤ Suggest a MedicAlert bracelet.
➤ Patients must be referred to St James's University Hospital MH investigation unit in Leeds, where a muscle biopsy will be taken for 'in vitro muscle contracture testing' (muscle tissue is exposed to caffeine and halothane which reduce the threshold for muscle contraction). This is the gold standard diagnostic test for MH.

CHAPTER 62

Needlestick injury

Needlestick injuries can have huge implications for the individual involved, not only in terms of disease transmission and employment effects but also because of the anxiety and psychological strain it can cause while waiting for test results. This question requires you to demonstrate knowledge on associated risk factors along with methods used to minimise these and explores your management of the situation, which should focus on ensuring the safety of both you and your patient using local guidelines.

You are suturing a central venous line in a 36-year-old male diagnosed with pancreatitis when you inadvertently sustain a needlestick injury. What immediate action would you take?

➤ Call for help so that someone can relieve you and look after the patient.
➤ Encourage free bleeding of the wound.
➤ Immediately wash the wound with soap and water (do not scrub or suck).
➤ Follow local policy and inform occupational health to report the incident and to seek further advice (out of hours go to your A&E department).
➤ Establish whether you should start to take post-exposure prophylaxis (PEP) to HIV, by performing a risk assessment of the patient.

How would you perform a 'risk assessment' of your patient?

A risk assessment aims to identify those individuals who are more likely to be infected with HIV, hepatitis B (HBV) or hepatitis C (HCV). Transmission rates are 0.3% for HIV, 3% for HCV and 30% HBV.

Explain to the patient what has happened and that for your safety, a formal risk-assessment is very important.

Ensure that this is done in private with no friends or family present.

➤ **History:**
  • HIV, HBV and HCV status
  • Sexuality: homosexual intercourse or casual partners including prostitutes
  • Use of intravenous drugs and needle sharing
  • Tattoos
  • Blood transfusions abroad or multiple blood transfusions
  • History of jaundice
  • Recent holiday or residency in a country with a high HIV incidence.
➤ **Examination:**
  • Tattoos
  • Needle track marks
  • Lymphadenopathy.
➤ **Investigations:** Gain the patient's consent to take blood for HIV, HBV and HCV testing (the patient must be given appropriate counselling prior to this – follow your local hospital protocol on 'donor' counselling).

What further steps would you undertake?

➤ Have your blood taken shortly after the injury to confirm your current status (follow-up blood tests will be required later).

➤ Commence post-exposure prophylaxis (PEP) if patient deemed to be high-risk. This should be ideally started within 1 hour of injury, and consists of a triple therapy regime of zidovudine, lamivudine and indinavir that is taken for 4 weeks. Unfortunately, these agents can cause serious side-effects such as jaundice, diabetes, vomiting and profound fatigue.

➤ Establish your hepatitis B status. All healthcare professionals should be vaccinated prior to starting work. If you are a known responder, you should be given a hepatitis B vaccine booster. If you are susceptible, you should be given an accelerated hepatitis B vaccination course along with hepatitis B immunoglobulin. There is currently no official treatment for suspected or confirmed exposure to hepatitis C.

➤ Inform your clinical lead, as a suspected exposure to HIV, HBV or HCV may preclude you from performing certain exposure-prone procedures. The Department of Health have stated airway manipulation using gloves is not an exposure prone procedure.

➤ Seek counselling.

➤ Complete a critical incident form.

What are the major risk factors associated with the transmission of blood-borne viruses?

➤ **Exposure to high-risk fluids:**
  • High-risk fluids: blood, amniotic, peritoneal, pleural, pericardial and cerebrospinal fluid, semen and vaginal secretions
  • Low-risk fluids: faeces, urine, saliva and vomit.

➤ **Mechanism of injury:**
  • Percutaneous injury (e.g. with needles)
  • Exposure of broken skin (e.g. cuts)
  • Exposure of mucous membrane (e.g. splash to the eye).

➤ **Type of instrument:** Hollow bore needles carry higher risk than solid needles.

➤ **Patient:** Blood or fluid from terminally ill patients or those with a high viral load is more contagious.

What precautions can be taken to reduce risk of infection?

➤ Universal precautions when performing any exposure-prone procedures: gloves, mask and goggles.

➤ Avoid resheathing needles and use sharps bin to dispose of equipment promptly.

➤ Cover open skin lesions (but ideally avoid patient contact).

➤ Avoid mouth-to-mouth ventilation.

➤ Use of HMEF filters on breathing circuits between patients.

➤ Hepatitis B vaccination of healthcare professionals.

➤ Exposure protection plan and management plan.

CHAPTER 63

ST segment changes

The ST segment of the ECG represents repolarisation of the ventricles. Changes in the appearance of the ST segments can be caused by myocardial ischaemia or myocardial infarction. In the face of ischaemia, ST segment depression or elevation may occur relative to the isoelectric line. Movement away from the isoelectric line of ≥ 1 mm is significant.

Intraoperative ST segment changes require rapid detection and management in order to correct and optimise coronary blood flow and reduce myocardial work. Intraoperatively, the commonest causes of myocardial ischaemia are rate-related ischaemia and hypotension.

How would you manage an anaesthetised patient with ST segment changes?

➤ **Immediate management:**
  - Give 100% oxygen.
  - Call for help and inform the surgeons of the need to conclude surgery as soon as possible.
  - Perform a rapid but thorough assessment of the patient, looking for precipitating causes, e.g. hypoxia, tachycardia, hypotension and acute blood loss. Address any correctable problems.
  - Ensure adequate coronary perfusion pressure (increase aortic diastolic pressure), optimise arterial oxygen content (increase FiO_2 and ensure normal Hb concentration), optimise coronary blood flow (increase diastolic time and promote coronary vasodilatation) and reduce myocardial oxygen consumption (reduce heart rate and force of contraction). Vasoactive drugs such as intravenous nitrates, β-blockers or vasopressors may be required.

➤ **Early management:**
  - Consider additional monitoring (arterial line and central line) if there seems to be physiological deterioration as a result of cardiac ischaemia.
  - Should the patient deteriorate further, e.g. refractory hypotension or pulmonary oedema, it would be sensible to use cardiac output monitoring devices if available (e.g. oesophageal Doppler or LiDCO). These should be used to guide fluid and inotropic therapy.

➤ **Post-operatively:**
  - Following the operation, transfer the patient to an area of high dependency care for observation and investigation.
  - Perform a 12-lead ECG, and if it is abnormal, continue to take serial ECGs.
  - Take blood for cardiac enzymes, U&Es and FBC and glucose.
  - After 12 hours, take blood for a troponin I level.
  - Request an urgent review by the cardiologists for ongoing management advice.
  - Document events clearly in the notes.

CHAPTER 64

Tachyarrhythmias

What are some of the causes of intraoperative tachyarrythmias?

➤ **Patient factors:** All patients undergoing anaesthesia and surgery are at risk of intraoperative arrhythmias. However, certain patients are at increased risk:
  - Pre-existing cardiac disease, e.g. ischaemic heart disease or valvular heart disease
  - Pre-existing arrhythmia, e.g. atrial fibrillation or Wolff–Parkinson–White syndrome
  - Pre-existing electrolyte disturbances, e.g. diuretic-induced hypokalaemia and hypomagnesaemia
  - Endocrine disease, e.g. thyrotoxicosis.

➤ **Anaesthetic factors:** General and regional anaesthetic techniques can have significant effects on cardiac function:
  - Drug-induced alteration in cardiac preload, contractility and afterload
  - Effects on coronary perfusion pressure
  - Effects on myocardial irritability
  - Effects on autonomic nervous system
  - Effects of hypoxia and hypercapnia
  - Electrolyte disturbances (either pre-existing or iatrogenic from fluid therapy)
  - Effects of intravascular devices (e.g. central venous lines) advanced too far and entering the right atrium.

➤ **Surgical factors:**
  - Effects of pneumoperitoneum related to laparoscopic surgery, e.g. vagal response, reduced venous return, fall in cardiac index or rise in SVR
  - Effects of hypercapnia related to laparoscopic surgery, e.g. arrhythmias
  - Effects of rapid fluid shifts
  - Systemic inflammatory response syndrome (SIRS) induced by tissue trauma.

  The combination of patient, anaesthetic and surgical factors may lead to the development of intraoperative arrhythmias. The arrhythmias may be benign (e.g. occasional ventricular ectopics) or potentially malignant arrhythmias may develop (e.g. ventricular tachycardia).

Describe your management of an intraoperative tachyarrhythmia

Management of intraoperative tachyarrhythmia follows general principles applicable to all tachyarrhythmia and specific treatments for certain types of tachyarrhythmia.

General management principles:

➤ Consider calling for assistance depending on the haemodynamic consequences of the arrhythmia.
➤ Diagnose the arrhythmia and establish the haemodynamic consequences – check blood pressure and end-tidal CO_2.
➤ Attempt to identify and treat the cause of the arrhythmia, e.g. adjust CVP line tip position or correct electrolyte disturbances.

➤ Attempt to maximise myocardial oxygen delivery by maintaining arterial oxygen content and coronary perfusion pressure.

➤ Check and correct electrolyte disturbances (potassium and magnesium): arterial blood gas analysis is the fastest method of obtaining potassium concentration (if hypokalaemia is present, in the majority of cases hypomagnesaemia will also be present).

➤ Attempt to correct any identified acid-base abnormalities detected on arterial blood gas.

Specific management:

➤ **Broad complex tachycardia (VF/VT/SVT with aberrant conduction)**
- If there is no pulse follow ALS protocol.
- If there is a pulse assess the haemodynamic consequences:
- **Systolic < 90 mmHg/heart rate > 150:** Synchronised DC cardioversion (up to 3 shocks). If refractory consider amiodarone 150 mg over 10 minutes followed by 300 mg over 1 hour and repeat shock if necessary. Consider lignocaine and overdrive pacing.
- **Systolic > 90 mmHg/heart rate < 150:** Correct K^+ (> 4.0 mmol/L) and Mg^{2+} (> 1.0 mmol/L). Administer amiodarone 150 mg IV over 10 minutes or lignocaine 50 mg over 2 minutes repeated every 5 minutes up to a total dose of 200 mg.

➤ **Narrow complex tachycardia (SVT/atrial flutter)**
- If there is no pulse follow the ALS protocol.
- If the rhythm is atrial fibrillation (AF), follow AF algorithm.
- If there is a pulse and atrial fibrillation is excluded assess the haemodynamic consequences:
- **Systolic < 90 mmHg/ventricular rate > 200:** Synchronised DC cardioversion (up to 3 shocks). Consider amiodarone 150 mg over 10 minutes followed by 300 mg over 1 hour and repeat shock if necessary.
- **Systolic > 90 mmHg/ventricular rate < 200:** Attempt vagal manoeuvre (e.g. carotid sinus massage). Consider adenosine boluses 6 mg, followed by up to three 12 mg doses. If resistant, consider use of esmolol, amiodarone, digoxin or verapamil.

➤ **Atrial fibrillation**

Management depends on the time of onset (i.e. acute/chronic AF and subsequent risk of systemic embolisation if sinus rhythm is restored), ventricular rate and the haemodynamic consequences:

Critical AF, ventricular rate > 150, hypotension and impaired perfusion

➤ Heparise if feasible (note risk of intraoperative bleeding)

➤ Administer synchronised DC cardioversion

➤ Administer amiodarone 300 mg IV over 1 hour followed by 900 mg over the following 23 hours

Intermediate AF, ventricular rate 100–150

If associated with haemodynamic compromise:

➤ Onset < 24 hours: Heparinise and administer synchronised DC cardioversion. Consider amiodarone IV 300 mg over 1 hour.

➤ Onset > 24 hours: Control rate initially with amiodarone IV 300 mg over 1 hour. Heparinise and later perform synchronised DC cardioversion.

If associated with normal haemodynamics:

➤ Onset < 24 hours: Heparinise and administer amiodarone IV 300 mg over 1 hour. Consider flecainide. Synchronised DC cardioversion may be required.

➤ Onset > 24 hours: Control rate initially with digoxin, verapamil or β-blockers. Heparinise and later perform synchronised DC cardioversion.

Low-risk AF, ventricular Rate < 100 with good perfusion

➤ Onset < 24 hours: Heparinise and administer amiodarone IV 300 mg over 1 hour. Consider flecanide.

➤ Onset > 24 hours: Heparinise and then later perform synchronised DC cardioversion.

Post-operative:

All patients who have suffered significant intraoperative arrhythmias should have cardiac monitoring in the initial post-operative period (including 12-lead ECG) and relevant cardiac follow-up if indicated.

ALS protocols have not been covered here but are likely to be examined in the OSCE.

CHAPTER 65

Venous air embolism (VAE)

VAE is a potential complication of many surgical procedures. The clinical features range from sub-clinical to life-threatening cardiovascular collapse depending upon the rate and volume of gas that is entrained into the circulation.

Examiners will expect an understanding of the types of procedures that are associated with an increased risk of VAE, and also the ability to diagnose and manage the problem.

What procedures are associated with a high risk of VAE?
➤ Neurosurgery, particularly surgery in the sitting position and surgery involving the cranium and dura
➤ Laparoscopic surgery with risk of direct intravascular gas insufflation
➤ Head and neck surgery with large areas of tissue exposed, often with vessels at subatmospheric pressure
➤ Orthopaedic surgery, e.g. polytrauma, cementing and reaming in long bone surgery
➤ Insertion of intravascular devices, e.g. central venous cannulation.

How can you diagnose VAE?
Symptoms and signs are primarily those of cardiovascular collapse (hypotension, tachy-cardia, arrhythmias and arterial desaturation) caused by the air embolus acting as an intracardiac air lock. In the correct clinical setting, suspicion for VAE must always remain high. In certain high-risk procedures (e.g. neurosurgery in the sitting position) monitoring should be used electively to aid early VAE detection and may include the following:
➤ Listen for audible hissing as gas enters the circulation.
➤ ECG: VAE is associated with an increase in pulmonary vascular resistance and the development of right ventricular dysfunction causing arrhythmias and possibly a right ventricular strain pattern.
➤ Capnography: Fall in end-tidal CO_2.
➤ CVP increases.
➤ Precordial stethoscope: Classic 'millwheel murmur'. This is insensitive and a late sign.
➤ Pulmonary artery pressure increases.
➤ Oesophageal Doppler is extremely useful in early detection of VAE.
➤ Transoesophageal echocardiography (TOE): Possibly the gold standard. Allows localisation of air to a specific cardiac chamber while enabling assessment of cardiac function.

What is the management of a suspected VAE?
State that this is an anaesthetic emergency and that you would call for senior anaesthetic assistance.
➤ Inform the surgeon who may be able to prevent further embolisation by compression of the surgical site or flooding the surgical site with saline.
➤ Administer 100% oxygen and discontinue nitrous oxide, which will increase bubble size due to its high solubility.

➤ Increase CVP by tilting the patient slightly head-down, administer fluid and increase PEEP.

➤ Position patient in left lateral head-down position if feasible, this may prevent embolisation into the pulmonary artery. In this position consider attempting to aspirate the air via a CVP line.

➤ Cardiovascular support with fluid and inotropic support may be required. CPR may also become necessary if the situation deteriorates.

➤ Terminate surgery as soon as safely possible.

➤ Arrange appropriate post-operative care (ITU or HDU).

➤ Document events when safely possible and complete a critical incident form.

➤ Explain event to the patient when possible.

Index

Entries in **bold** denote tables and figures